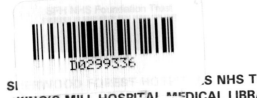
Continence: Promotion and Management by the Primary Health Care Team

Consensus Guidelines

Continence: Promotion and Management by the Primary Health Care Team

Consensus Guidelines

Denise Button, Brenda Roe, Christine Webb,
Tony Frith, David Colin-Thome and Lance Gardner

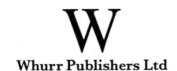

Whurr Publishers Ltd

© 1998 Whurr Publishers Ltd
First published 1998 by
Whurr Publishers Ltd
19B Compton Terrace, London N1 2UN, England

Reprinted 1999

British Library Cataloguing in Publication Data
A catalogue record for this book is available from the
British Library.

ISBN 1 86156 078 8

Printed and bound in the UK by Athenaeum Press Ltd,
Gateshead, Tyne & Wear

Contents

Foreword

The Castlefields Practice in Runcorn has a well established health needs assessment process. This publication is the outcome of a process in which primary health care workers identified a clinical need in relation to incontinence. The clinical staff expressed dissatisfaction about the quality of care offered to this group of patients, and this was reinforced by patient feedback.

Members of the practice were aware that the National Health Services Executive (NHSE) was simultaneously actively facilitating guideline development across the NHS. Traditionally such initiatives tended to be undertaken in a secondary care setting. However, the subject material, the context of a Primary Care Led NHS and the assertiveness of our team led us to bid for a primary care-focused clinical guideline initiative. This provided the resources for a project manager/facilitator to utilise an evidence-based approach in the development of these guidelines, involving both a systematic review of the research evidence and a consensus conference. We are deeply indebted to Brenda Roe and Christine Webb for helping us to move from simply identifying a problem to active involvement, and to Denise Button for being an excellent project manager/facilitator. Her critical appraisal research skills and her ability to empower us were immense. Well deserved thanks are also due to all the experts and consumer representatives involved, to our motivated Primary Health Care Team and especially to our patients who were involved in the subsequent implementation and evaluation of the guidelines and who I confidently expect to benefit from this work.

A key task at the practice is to ensure that the guidelines continue as a working document, rather than being consigned to a filing system, thereby ensuring continuing quality care. We are confident that we will continue to deliver a quality agenda but realise that audit must be an imperative.

Given the continuing importance of primary care within the current health service provision, I feel this publication is timely and topical, but its greatest importance is in enabling good care to be delivered to a group of patients often previously unrecognised.

David Colin-Thome
General Practitioner, Castlefields Health Centre, Runcorn;
Senior Medical Officer (Part-time) NHSME, Scottish Office; Fellow,
Health Services Management Unit, University of Manchester.

The authors

Denise Button BSc(Hons), MSc, RN, RNT, Postgraduate student, School of Nursing Studies, University of Manchester. Formerly Project Officer, Castlefields Health Centre, Runcorn, Cheshire.

Brenda Roe PhD, RN, FRSH, Honorary Senior Research Fellow, Institute of Human Ageing, University of Liverpool. Formerly Senior Research Fellow, Health Services Research Unit, University of Oxford.

Christine Webb BA(Hons), MSc, PhD, RN, RSCN, RNT, Professor of Health Studies, Institute of Health Studies, University of Plymouth. Formerly Professor of Nursing, School of Nursing Studies, University of Manchester.

Tony Frith MB, ChB, MRCGP, General Practitioner, Castlefields Health Centre, Runcorn, Cheshire.

David Colin-Thome MB, BS, FRCGP, D(Obst)RCOG, DCH, (Hon)MFPHM, General Practitioner, Castlefields Health Centre, Runcorn, Cheshire.

Lance Gardner MSc, RN, RHV, NPDip, Professional Development Officer, Queens Nursing Institute and Salford Community Health Care NHS Trust. Formerly Business/General Manager and Nurse Practitioner, Castlefields Health Centre, Runcorn, Cheshire.

Acknowledgements

The project team would like to acknowledge the support and assistance received during the development of these guidelines from the NHS Executive. In particular; Dr Karin von Degenberg, Professor Michael Deighan, Ms Debra Humphris, Ms Mary Edwards and Mr Tom Keighley.

The project team are grateful to the following people and organisations who have contributed to the development of the guidelines either as members of the Expert Panel or during the consultation phase.

Conference expert panel (As at January 1995)

Dr James Barrett
Consultant Physician for the
Elderly, Clatterbridge Hospital,
Wirral

Professor John Brocklehurst
Associate Director, Research
Unit, Royal College of Physicians

Ms Pam Brookfield
Continence Adviser, specialist
in care of children with enuresis, Cheshire Community
Healthcare Trust

Ms Bunny Brown
Senior Physiotherapist, Halton
General Hospital NHS Trust

Miss Millie Carter
Nursing Officer, Department of
Health

Professor C.M. Castleden
Professor of Medicine for the
Elderly, Leicester General
Hospital

Dr Francine Cheater
Senior Lecturer in Clinical
Audit (Nursing), Eli Lilly
National Clinical Audit Centre

Ms Helen Crew
District Nurse, Castlefields
Health Centre

Ms Sylvia Critchley
Practice Nurse, Castlefields
Health Centre

Ms Jeanette Haslam
Senior Physiotherapist Chorley,
Lancs.

Mr Paul Hilton
Consultant Gynaecologist,
Subspecialist in Urogynaecol-
ogy, Royal Victoria Hospital,
Newcastle

Dr Sue Hope
General Practitioner, G.P.
Member of working group on
female incontinence, Oxford

Mr Ed Kiff
Consultant Surgeon, Withington
Hospital, South Manchester

Dr Jo Laycock
Urotherapy Manager/Research
Physiotherapist, Bradford Royal
Infirmary

Ms Jane Pattison
Senior Lecturer, Liverpool John
Moores University/School of
Health Care Studies, Whiston
Hospital

Ms Marilyn Simms
Health Visitor, Castlefields
Health Centre

Mr Mark Stott
Consultant Surgeon, Exeter

Mr John Sutherst
Consultant Gynaecologist,
Arrowe Park Hospital, Wirral

Ms Kate Williams
Research and Development
Officer, National Institute of
Nursing, Radcliffe Infirmary,
Oxford

Ms Ann Winder
District Continence Adviser,
Bristol

Organisation representatives on the panel

Ms Wendy Colley
Chair, Association for Conti-
nence Advice/Continence
Adviser, Cumbria

Ms Christine Norton
Director, The Continence
Foundation

Ms Hilary Oliver
Chair RCN Continence
Forum/Nurse Manager
Bradford Community Trust

Consumer/self-help group representatives on the panel

Mr Stephen Hunt
General Manager, Children's
Services, Hinchingbrook
Health Centre Trust, Represen-
tative for Enuresis Resource and
Information Centre (ERIC),
Bristol

Ms Laurel Salthouse
Secretary INCONTACT –
National Action on Incontinence

Mr Colin Turner
Full Time Carer representing
Halton Carer's Forum

Contributors

The following individuals and organisations have been involved
through the process of consultation. They were invited to comment
on the second draft of the guideline document and many provided
valuable feedback and comments.

Mr Paul Abrams
Consultant Urologist, Hon.
Secretary, International Conti-
nence Society

Dr David Bainton
Hon. Consultant in Public
Health Medicine, Gwent
Health Commission

Mr Yogesh Chadha
Health Services Research Unit,
Aberdeen

Ms Jane Clayton
Social Policy Research Unit,
York University

Ms Kiki de Courcy-Ireland
Continence Adviser, Ealing
Hammersmith and Hounslow
Health Agency

Ms Penny Dobson
Director, Enuresis Resource and
Information Centre (ERIC)

Dr D.S. Memel
General Practitioner, Bristol

Mr Richard Walsh
Department of Health

Amalgamated School Nurses'
Association

British Association of Urological
Surgeons

British Geriatrics Society for
Health in Old Age

British Paediatric Association

Health Visitors' Association

Queen's Nursing Institute

Royal College of General
Practitioners

Royal College of Midwifery

Royal College of Nursing

Royal College of Physicians

Royal College of Obstetricians
and Gynaecologists

Royal College of Surgeons

Chapter 1
Introduction and background

Background

In 1993 the NHS Executive Nursing Directorate invited suggestions from various centres of excellence, Trusts and health care organisations for clinical areas that would benefit from the development of clinical guidelines. This was in relation to the achievement of target 3 of the government's *A Vision for the Future* (DH, 1993), which stressed the need for clinical protocols.

The promotion and management of continence met the criteria identified by the NHS Executive for the development of guidelines as follows.

Common condition/high cost of care

Incontinence is a widespread problem affecting all age groups, the nature of which is complex. Whilst studies have produced varying prevalence figures for urinary and faecal incontinence (Mohide, 1992; Barrett, 1993), the estimate made by Smith in 1982 of at least three million adult sufferers in the United Kingdom remains sound. However, these are conditions which may go largely undetected in the community (Thomas *et al.*, 1980; Jolleys, 1988; O'Brien *et al.*, 1991; Brocklehurst, 1993). Individuals with both urinary and faecal incontinence continue to be seen and cared for by the members of the Primary Health Care Team (PHCT) as well as specialist continence services, subject to their availability.

Purchasers of continence care (either health authority or fund-holding GP practices) often do so by arranging block contracts with the community nursing services. Continence care is therefore neither discreet nor specific and tends to be grouped in with all other aspects of community nursing. The cost to the NHS of providing continence aids and appliances to sufferers has been estimated to be at least £50 million per annum in the United Kingdom (DH, 1991).

Existence of a sound knowledge base

A sizeable volume of literature and research exists on the subject of urinary incontinence. It has been argued that health care costs could be reduced through the implementation of the research findings (AHCPR, 1992). Similarly, the implementation of the research findings on faecal incontinence, although less in volume, may also improve health care for sufferers (Roe, 1992a).

Professional interest and public concern

Professional and political interest in continence services are evident through the high profile they have recently achieved in the NHS's Management Executive planning and priorities guidelines for 1994/95 (NHSME, 1993). The initiation by the Department of Health of a first National Continence Week in March 1994, followed in 1995 by a Continence Awareness Day, is also indicative of the importance of this subject in current health care and has served to raise public interest and concern.

Consequently, the promotion and management of continence by the PHCT was included as part of the NHS Executive Consensus Strategy for Major Clinical Guidelines.

Methodology

The guidelines were produced using a systematic review of the literature and a multidisciplinary consensus conference of approximately 30 invited experts and clinicians in continence care and consumers of continence services. Consensus statements produced during the conference were cross-referenced with the literature review to provide supporting rationales.

In this way, national clinical guidelines were produced which could subsequently be translated into local guidelines by purchasers and providers.

The methodology used for the systematic review of the literature is outlined in Chapter 4, and Appendix III describes the overall methodology.

Aims of the guidelines

The guidelines are intended to:

1. Be used by **all members** of the PHCT.
2. Provide principles of good practice for the PHCT, which are evidence based wherever possible, in the care of individuals of all ages suffering from urinary incontinence (including enuresis in children) and faecal incontinence.

   Where there are specific areas of concern for different types of incontinence or age groups, these are identified. The guidelines do not focus on the use of specific surgical techniques, since this is not within the remit of the PHCT. The treatment of extraurethral urinary incontinence is not dealt with by these guidelines.
3. Give examples of good practice and other national clinical guidelines which may be of use to health care professionals and which have been referred to in the development of these guidelines (Appendix I). These include the Charter for Continence and the Charter for Children with Bedwetting and Daytime Wetting and their Families, which were recently produced for consumers of continence services by relevant organisations and consumer groups.
4. Make recommendations for further research and development in relation to the promotion and management of continence, identified from both the literature review and the consensus conference.
5. Be interpreted and implemented locally by each PHCT, taking account of local requirements.

A summary of the guideline statements is given in order to provide an overview of the whole of the guidelines. It is not intended that the statements be used in isolation from the supporting rationales, since these provide the evidence for the guidelines.

Implementation and evaluation

The guidelines have initially been implemented and evaluated at Castlefields Health Centre, Runcorn (Button *et al.*, 1996). Further pilot sites will then be determined for subsequent implementation and evaluation.

The guidelines will be subject to review in the future, in line with health care developments.

Chapter 2
Summary of guideline statements

Definition of incontinence

- Incontinence is 'a condition where involuntary loss of urine or faeces is a social or hygienic problem'.

The role of the primary health care team in the promotion and management of continence

- Incontinence is common amongst individuals in the community and can in many cases be treated by members of the PHCT.
- All members of the PHCT should have an awareness of the problems of incontinence, but there should be at least one member with the appropriate knowledge and expertise to undertake an assessment, diagnose and treat incontinence.
- The GP should be involved at an appropriate stage in the decision-making process.
- There should be an agreed, consistent approach within the PHCT to the care of individuals with incontinence.

Individuals'/carers' involvement in their care

- Everyone has a right to have their incontinence assessed and treated by a health care professional who has the appropriate knowledge and expertise.
- The individual has a right to be treated by a member of the PHCT before secondary referral if appropriate.

5

- Individuals and carers have a right to be involved in the decision-making process about their care and to have an awareness of the options available.
- Individuals in nursing and residential homes should receive the same standard of care as those in their own homes.

Screening/identification

- Identification of incontinent people in high-risk groups should be undertaken by the PHCT.
- The PHCT should utilise opportunities for increasing public awareness of the problem of incontinence.

Assessment

- The initial contact by any member of the PHCT with the person suffering from incontinence is crucial to the success of future care.
- The assessment should be undertaken by a health care professional who has the appropriate knowledge and expertise.
- There should be a single assessment tool that is usable by all members of the PHCT and which follows the individual.
- The assessment should take account of the whole person and include sufficient information to lead to a working diagnosis and exclude/identify other diseases and contributory factors.

Promotion/restoration of continence

- Restoration of continence should be the primary aim of care for all individuals.
- Contributory factors should be addressed before other interventions are undertaken.
- In many cases, a therapeutic trial in a primary care setting should precede secondary care. Referral to secondary care is necessary in certain specific circumstances.
- The PHCT should have knowledge of available specialist skills to enable appropriate referral.
- Behavioural techniques may be used successfully by knowledgeable staff to restore or improve continence in some cases. These include:
  - bladder re-education programmes;
  - conditioning methods;
  - pelvic floor re-education;
  - biofeedback.

- Drugs should generally be used in conjunction with other therapy after contributory factors have been addressed.
- Regardless of the drug chosen, the initial dose should be relatively low and be titrated to balance the side-effects with efficacy.
- The PHCT should ensure the education, motivation and support of the individual/carer as this is vital to the success of any treatment.
- The progress of the individual should be reassessed regularly at appropriate time intervals.
- All treatments for the restoration of continence should be undertaken by appropriately trained personnel, should conform to preset standards and should be subject to audit.

Management of incontinence

- The restoration of continence should be the aim for all persons. The management of incontinence using aids and appliances should only occur either concurrently with strategies for the restoration of continence or when such strategies have been shown to fail.
- No aid or appliance should be issued without an assessment of need by an appropriately trained health care professional.
- The choice of the individual should be a key consideration in the determination of the management approach and the selection of products.
- The PHCT should ensure that the individual/carer is adequately educated about the correct use of any aid or appliance issued.
- All individuals should be regularly reviewed, as their needs may change and/or new management approaches may become available.

Prevention

- Opportunities for the prevention of incontinence should be considered by the PHCT.

Educational issues

- Each PHCT should have an educational strategy that aims to increase the awareness of all members of the problems of incontinence.
- There should be opportunities, if necessary, for at least one member of the PHCT to undergo additional training to increase their levels of knowledge and expertise in relation to incontinence.

Continuous quality improvement

- There should be nationally agreed standards for the provision of continence care by the PHCT.
- There should be a continuous quality improvement programme for the service offered by the PHCT to sufferers of incontinence, which should include as a minimum:
    - clinical audit using locally agreed outcome measures;
    - audit of the educational strategy;
    - audit of the knowledge and commitment of members of the PHCT to the guideline;
    - the appraisal of consumer views.
- There should be continuous quality improvement of these guidelines, through regular review and revision as appropriate.

Chapter 3
Guidelines

Definition of incontinence

- **Incontinence is 'a condition where involuntary loss of urine or faeces is a social or hygienic problem'.**

Rationale

This definition was approved by the consensus panel and is an adaptation of the International Continence Society (ICS) definition of urinary incontinence (Andersen *et al.*, 1988). The ICS definition requires the objective demonstration of incontinence; however, the panel agreed that this was neither necessary nor possible in a primary health care setting.

The agreed definition acknowledges the social and hygienic aspects of incontinence and that incontinence (which includes enuresis in children) is a problem to the individual and/or carer if they say it is.

Whilst this definition is broad and encompasses many types of incontinence, these guidelines do not cover urinary incontinence arising from extraurethral loss of urine or incontinence due to congenital problems of the urinary or gastrointestinal tract.

For the purpose of these guidelines, the following definition for enuresis in children, recommended by the Enuresis Resource and Information Centre (ERIC), has been used (Forsythe and Butler, 1989).

> The involuntary discharge of urine by day or night or both, in a child aged five years or older, in the absence of congenital or acquired defects of the nervous system or urinary tract.

9

The role of the primary health care team in the promotion and management of continence

- **Incontinence is common amongst individuals in the community and can in many cases be treated by members of the PHCT.**

Rationale

Prevalence studies are difficult to compare. However, the following prevalence rates for urinary incontinence have been found in men:

- 1.6–6.6% for men aged over 15 years;
- 7–10% for men over 55 years.

Urinary incontinence is more common in women:

- at least 8% report of some urinary incontinence before the age of 65.
- between 12% and 25% of women aged over 65 years are affected.

In addition, 1% of adults are reported to have nocturnal enuresis, i.e. bedwetting at night (Thomas *et al.*, 1980; O'Brien *et al.*, 1991; Brocklehurst, 1993; Molander, 1993).

Nocturnal enuresis in children is also reported in:

- 15% of children aged 5 years (Clark *et al.*, 1994);
- 7% of boys and 3% of girls aged 7 years (Hellstrom *et al.*, 1990b);
- 6.2% of boys and 3.5% of girls aged 11–12 years (Swithinbank *et al.*, 1994).

Day- and night-time wetting occurs in 2–10% of schoolchildren (Hellstrom *et al.*, 1990b; Bloom *et al.*, 1993). However, 15–16% of children who bedwet experience spontaneous remission each year (Clark *et al.*, 1994).

Faecal incontinence also affects all age groups but is most common in elderly people. Prevalence studies suggest that fewer than 4 people per 1000 of the population aged 15–64 years suffer from faecal incontinence but that this rises after the age of 65 years to 11 per 1000 for men and 13.3 per 1000 for women (Thomas *et al.*, 1984). Both urinary and faecal incontinence are more common in elderly people in institutional care.

Studies have shown that many cases of urinary incontinence can be treated effectively by the PHCT, without referral to secondary care (O'Brien *et al.*, 1991; Lagro-Janssen, Debruyne, Smits *et al.*, 1992; Harrison and Memel, 1994). The effective treatment of faecal incontinence in many individuals, especially in elderly people, is also possible by the PHCT (Barrett, 1992).

- **All members of the PHCT should have an awareness of the problems of incontinence, but there should be at least one member with the appropriate knowledge and expertise to undertake an assessment, diagnose and treat incontinence.**

Rationale

There was consensus that, as incontinence is such a common problem in the community, it is essential that all members of the PHCT have a basic understanding of the condition and that successful treatment is in many cases possible.

The assessment, diagnosis and treatment of an individual with incontinence requires additional knowledge and expertise. Members of the PHCT should know who, within the team, has this expertise or where this expertise can be accessed, and be able to refer individuals to them for further assessment and care as appropriate.

- **The GP should be involved at an appropriate stage in the decision-making process.**

Rationale

The panel thought it important that the GP should always be involved at some stage of the decision-making process about each individual's care. However, it may not always be the GP who has the knowledge and expertise to assess, treat and manage an individual with incontinence. Each PHCT should therefore determine what form the GP's involvement will take and at what stage in an individual's care it will occur, which may well vary between cases.

- **There should be an agreed, consistent approach within the PHCT to the care of individuals with incontinence.**

Rationale

There was consensus within the panel that the PHCT should determine a local policy for the promotion and restoration of continence and the management of incontinence. This should help to ensure that individuals receive consistent advice from health care professionals, which may in turn help to increase the success of treatment. In the case of children suffering from enuresis, it is essential that one member of the team is responsible for that care in order to maintain consistency, thereby maximising the success rate and reducing drop-out rates (Clark *et al.*, 1994).

Individuals'/carers' involvement in their care

- **Everyone has a right to have their incontinence assessed and treated by a health care professional who has the appropriate knowledge and expertise.**

Rationale

A full assessment is essential for all individuals reporting continence problems, as treatment is dependent upon the cause or causes (Resnick, 1990a, 1990b; Brocklehurst, 1990a; Barrett, 1992; Duffin, 1992; Morgan, 1993; Clark *et al.*, 1994). The individual and/or their carer is entitled to expect a full assessment to be undertaken, and they should be seen as partners in the assessment process (Charter for Continence, 1995; ERIC, 1995; NHSE, 1995).

- **The individual has a right to be treated by a member of the PHCT before secondary referral if appropriate.**

Rationale

There was consensus that care should be provided initially within the primary care setting if possible and appropriate. It was felt that most individuals would prefer to be treated by the PHCT if possible, since (1) they would already be familiar with them and (2) secondary care requiring hospital or clinic visits may involve financial costs and inconvenience to the individual and/or carer.

- **Individuals and carers have a right to be involved in the decision-making process about their care and to have an awareness of the options available.**

Rationale

The advantages and disadvantages of the various treatment and management options should be explained to individuals and/or carers by the PHCT, including details of risks and side-effects where necessary, in order to enable informed decisions to be taken (Charter for Continence, 1995; ERIC, 1995; DH, 1995).

- **Individuals in nursing and residential homes should receive the same standard of care as those in their own homes.**

Rationale

The prevalence of both urinary and faecal incontinence is greater in institutional care than in the general community (Barrett, 1992; Davidson and Borrie, 1992; Ouslander, 1993). There was consensus that residents of nursing and residential homes have the right to care equivalent to that of individuals in their own homes, and that the PHCT should help to ensure this.

Screening/identification

- **The identification of incontinent people in high risk groups should be undertaken by the PHCT.**

Rationale

Incontinence is a distressing problem, yet some people do not consult their doctors about the complaint. This is very often because people think that it is 'a normal part of ageing' or 'a usual woman's complaint', or that 'nothing can be done'; others are too embarrassed to ask for help (Jolleys, 1988; Devlin, 1991; O'Brien *et al.*, 1991; Barrett, 1992; Goldstein *et al.*, 1992; Hunskaar, 1992; Brocklehurst, 1993; Harrison and Memel, 1994).

Urinary incontinence is known to be more common in elderly people and in women who have had children. Faecal incontinence also occurs more often in these two groups. Enuresis, particularly nocturnal enuresis, is fairly common in schoolage children.

As people may be reluctant to ask for help, the PHCT should use opportunities to identify these individuals and to offer help and advice. Postnatal checks, over 75-year-olds' screening, Well Man/Woman clinics, cervical cytology screening and school medicals present such opportunities. Questions on bowel and bladder problems should be an integral part of each of these.

- **The PHCT should utilise opportunities for increasing public awareness about the problem of incontinence.**

Rationale

The public are often unaware of how common incontinence is and that it can be treated (Goldstein *et al.*, 1992; Brocklehurst, 1993;

Harrison and Memel, 1994; Reymart and Hunskarr, 1994). There was consensus that opportunities that may be used by the PHCT to increase awareness include the screening situations outlined earlier. Providing leaflets, posters and details of self-help groups in doctors' surgeries/clinics may help. Addresses of self-help groups and useful organisations are given in Appendix II.

Assessment

- **The initial contact by any member of the PHCT with the person suffering from incontinence is crucial to the success of future care.**

Rationale

Since incontinence can be an embarrassing condition, individuals may have been reluctant to discuss their problem with their doctor, some not even mentioning it to their spouses. Many sufferers of incontinence, as well as parents of children with enuresis, have waited a long time before eventually approaching a health care professional (Jolleys, 1988; Devlin, 1991; Goldstein *et al.*, 1992; Brocklehurst, 1993; Reymart and Hunskaar, 1994). It is therefore vital that when the person does first present to the PHCT, the condition is acknowledged and dealt with sensitively and seriously. A positive and supportive approach is vital from the beginning.

In the case of children, reassurance should be given to both parent and child by explaining the prevalence figures and that wetting or bedwetting is not under the child's control (i.e. is not due to laziness or a lack of willpower). A supportive relationship between health care professional and parent and child has been shown to be a factor in the successful treatment of enuresis (Clark *et al.*, 1994).

Referring individuals and/or carers to self-help groups may be useful for further information and support. Addresses are given in Appendix II.

- **The assessment should be undertaken by a health care pro-fessional who has the appropriate knowledge and expertise.**

Rationale

The person suffering from incontinence may present to any member of the PHCT. That member of the team should acknowledge the problem in a supportive way but then refer the individual for a more detailed assessment to the health care professional within the team who has the appropriate knowledge and expertise (Morgan, 1993; Charter for Continence, 1995; DH, 1995; ERIC, 1995).

- **There should be a single assessment tool that is usable by all members of the PHCT and which follows the individual.**

Rationale

There was consensus that, as the person with incontinence may be seen by more than one member of the PHCT, the use of a single assessment tool should avoid unnecessary repetition of information and examination and improve consistency of care. The assessment tool should, however, meet the requirements of all health professionals who may use it and be compatible with the record-keeping systems in place. The Enuresis Resource and Information Centre (ERIC) have produced a resource pack that includes assessment forms for children (Butler, 1993).

- **The assessment should take account of the whole person and include sufficient information to lead to a working diagnosis and exclude/identify other diseases and contributory factors.**

Rationale

The impact of incontinence on individuals and/or their carers has been shown to affect their quality of life as well as their physical functioning, including effects on social activity, sexual activity and psychological state (Walters *et al.*, 1990; Dowd, 1991; Thomas and Morse, 1991; Lagro-Janssen, Smits *et al.*, 1992; Ashworth and Hagan, 1993; Brocklehurst, 1993; Grimby *et al.*, 1993). It is therefore important that an assessment, whilst identifying possible causes and contributory factors of the incontinence, also includes these other aspects and considers the whole person rather than just the condition. As a full assessment of an individual may take a while, it may be undertaken over a period of time.

The treatment of urinary and faecal incontinence is invariably related to cause, and the assessment should therefore identify possible causes and achieve a working diagnosis. The causes of urinary and faecal incontinence and enuresis are multifactorial, and several causes are very often involved in one case. Additionally, various factors indicate an increased likelihood of developing incontinence. The causes and risk factors are summarised below (Diokno *et al.*,

1990; Cheater, 1992; Barrett, 1992, 1993; Maizels *et al.*, 1993; Butler, 1994; Clark *et al.*, 1994):

Causes of urinary incontinence in adults

There may be various causes:

1. pathophysiological factors:
   * detrusor instability;
   * sphincter weakness, very often related to childbirth;
   * outflow obstruction;
   * the effects of neurological disease on the bladder;
2. factors affecting bladder function:
   * urinary tract infection;
   * faecal impaction;
   * drug therapy, including over-the-counter medications;
   * endocrine disorders;
   * effects of ageing on bladder function;
   * medical illnesses, e.g. cardiovascular problems and stroke;
   * intake of alcohol and caffeine;
3. factors affecting the ability to cope with the bladder:
   * mobility and physical functioning;
   * developmental factors, e.g. people with learning disabilities;
   * environmental factors, e.g. distance and access to the toilet;
   * mental state, e.g. dementia, depression or anxiety;
   * psychological factors, e.g. bereavement;
   * institutionalisation;
   * carers' attitudes and actions.

Urinary incontinence was found to be more likely to develop in adults when the following factors existed:

* a family history of childhood bedwetting (Moore *et al.*, 1991; Foldspang and Mommsen, 1994);
* pregnancy (Diokno *et al.*, 1990; Viktrup *et al.*, 1992);
* parity (Simeonova and Bengtsson, 1990; Foldspang *et al.*, 1992; Molander, 1993; Harrison and Memel, 1994);
* previous abdominal or urogynaecological surgery (Diokno *et al.*, 1990; Mommsen *et al.*, 1993).

Cause of urinary incontinence and enuresis in children

These may be:

1. pathophysiological factors:
   * detrusor instability;

- effects of neurological disease on the bladder;
- congenital anomaly;
- urinary tract infection;
2. associated factors
   - developmental factors, e.g. children with learning disabilities;
   - environmental factors, e.g. distance and access to the toilet, and bedtime routines.

Factors causing nocturnal enuresis in children

The aetiology of nocturnal enuresis in children remains unclear, and several factors have been implicated, although research evidence for some of these is contradictory and therefore inconclusive. The factors outlined below are those for which the research evidence was reasonably consistent:

- developmental factors, e.g. children with learning disabilities (Butler, 1994);
- environmental factors, e.g. distance and access to the toilet, and bedtime routines (Butler, 1994);
- urinary tract infection (Hansson 1992; Maizels *et al.*, 1993).

Additionally, the following factors indicated an increased likelihood of the development of nocturnal enuresis in children:

- genetic factors–a family history of childhood bedwetting (Rappaport, 1993);
- stressful events in early life (Devlin, 1991);
- in children from lower socio-economic classes and larger families living in overcrowded conditions (Butler, 1994).

Causes of faecal incontinence

Causes of faecal incontinence include:

- colorectal disease/diarrhoea;
- drugs, especially laxatives;
- anorectal incontinence (idiopathic), often involving weakness of the external and/or internal anal sphincters and pelvic floor muscles, which may be related to childbirth;
- faecal impaction, the most common cause in elderly people;
- faecal retention in children;
- neurological causes, including neurological disease involving the

pelvic floor and the central nervous system, dementia, unconsciousness and behavioural causes;
- immobility;
- developmental factors, e.g. learning difficulties.

Childbirth increases the likelihood of a woman developing faecal
incontinence (Barrett, 1993).

The assessment for a child aged 5–16 years with daytime wetting
or nocturnal enuresis is outlined in Table 3.1. More information on
the assessment of the child with enuresis is available from ERIC in
their *Guide to Enuresis* (published by Blackwell in 1995).

Table 3.2 shows the minimum assessment required of the adult
with urinary incontinence (Brocklehurst, 1990a; Resnick 1990a, b;
Duffin, 1992; Walters and Realini, 1992; Houston, 1993;
Bernard, 1994). Table 3.3 gives the minimum assessment for an
individual with faecal incontinence (Barrett, 1992, 1993; Bartolo
et al., 1994).

Table 3.1: Assessment by the PHCT of a child aged 5–16 with enuresis

---

History:
of the problem, including wetting characteristics, timing, amount and other urinary
symptoms
fluid intake, type, amount and timing
bowel control
environmental factors, e.g. bedroom access to toilet, bedtime routines
the child's attitude to the problem
family reaction, including parental attitudes
'functional pay-offs' when wetting occurs, e.g. sleeping in parents' bed, cuddle from
mother
education history
family history of enuresis
medical history

Physical examination, including:
weight, height, growth data, blood pressure
abdominal examination, palpable bladder, abnormal genitalia
neurological examination

Tests:
urinalysis
midstream urine for culture

Morgan, 1993; Rushton, 1993; Clark *et al.*, 1994. See also ERIC's *A Guide to Enuresis*,
published by Blackwell, 1995.

Table 3.2: Assessment of the adult with urinary incontinence

History:
symptoms of incontinence, characteristics, frequency, duration, onset, severity, precipitants, current methods of management
effects on quality of life on individual/carer, including effects on sexual activity
medical, surgical, neurological, genitourinary and obstetric history
review of all medications and smoking
functional abilities
environmental factors
developmental factors
fluid intake, amount and type
bowel function, including control of flatus
height, weight and body mass index
family history of urinary problems

Physical examination, including:
abdominal palpation
examination of perineum
pelvic examination and digital vaginal assessment in women
rectal examination in men and if indicated in women
general examination for neurological abnormalities or other precipitory causes
general mobility and physical functioning

Tests, including:
urinalysis
midstream urine for culture and sensitivity and presence of red cells
provocative stress test in women
estimation of post-voiding residual urine
completion of a frequency/volume chart

Brocklehurst, 1990a; Resnick, 1990a, b; Duffin, 1992; Walters and Realini, 1992; Houston, 1993; Bernard, 1994.

Table 3.3: Assessment of the individual with faecal incontinence

History:
incontinence symptoms, duration, onset, frequency, type of stool, current methods of management
effects on quality of life of individual/carer
defaecation history
fluid intake and dietary history
review of all medications
medical, neurological, surgical, gynaecological and obstetric history

Physical examination:
general mobility and physical functioning
neurological assessment
abdominal palpation
rectal examination
examination of perineum

Barrett, 1992, 1993; Bartolo *et al.*, 1994.

Promotion/restoration of continence

- **Restoration of continence should be the primary aim of care for all individuals.**

Rationale

Comparisons of studies that have demonstrated the effective treatment of incontinence through the promotion and restoration of continence cannot be made because of differences in methodology, sampling and outcome measures. However, it is possible to conclude that, in a large proportion of cases, both urinary and faecal continence can be restored or improved in both adults and children (Fantl *et al.*, 1991; Hyland, 1991; Mouritsen *et al.*, 1991; O'Brien *et al.*, 1991; Wells *et al.*, 1991; Barrett, 1992; Lagro-Janssen, Debruyne, Smits *et al.*, 1992; Elia *et al.*, 1993; Hahn *et al.*, 1993; Maizels *et al.*, 1993; Clark *et al.*, 1994; Harrison and Memel, 1994). This should therefore be the primary aim of care in all cases, including people with physical and/or learning disabilities.

- **Contributory factors should be addressed before other interventions are undertaken.**

Rationale

Various factors may contribute to the problem of incontinence, many of which can be addressed by the PHCT either before other treatments are commenced or concurrently with treatment or management of the problem. These factors include:

1. Urinary incontinence in adults–contributory factors:
   - smoking (Bump and McClish, 1992, 1994);
   - excessively high or low fluid intake (Cheater, 1992);
   - a high caffeine intake (Creighton and Stanton, 1990);
   - a high body mass index (Simeonova and Bengsten, 1990; Burgio *et al.*, 1991; Bump *et al.*, 1992);
   - atrophic vaginitis and hypo-oestrogenism (Molander, 1993);
   - other physical disabilities, e.g. arthritis.
2. Nocturnal enuresis in children–contributory factors:
   - upper airway obstruction (Weider *et al.*, 1991);
   - attitudes of the parent and/or child to the enuresis (Maizels *et al.*, 1993; Butler, 1994);
   - additionally, various factors that may predict a response to treatment for nocturnal enuresis in children are described by

Butler (1994) and summarised by Clark *et al.* (1994). These factors should be considered when treating such children.

3. Faecal incontinence–contributory factors:
   - fluid and dietary intake, especially very high or low fibre intake;
   - inappropriate use of laxatives;
   - medications;
   - inappropriate toileting habits, especially in children;
   - other physical disability, e.g. arthritis (Barrett, 1992, 1993).

Addressing such contributory factors may result in an improvement of both faecal and urinary continence without the need for further intervention, or may at least assist in the restoration of continence in conjunction with other therapy.

- **Referral:**
  In many cases a therapeutic trial in a primary care setting should precede secondary care. Referral to secondary care is necessary in certain specific circumstances.

Rationale

There was consensus that a working diagnosis should be achieved by the PHCT in most cases. A therapeutic trial using behavioural techniques and/or possibly drug therapy in a primary health care setting should then be possible in many cases (Jolleys, 1988; Brocklehurst, 1990a; Resnick, 1990a; Lagro-Janssen, Debruyne, Smits *et al.*, 1991; O'Brien *et al.*, 1991; Barrett, 1992; Walters and Realini, 1992; Houston, 1993; Bernard, 1994; Harrison and Memel, 1994). Referral to specialist secondary care for further investigation, surgery, specialist advice or treatment is required immediately in circumstances where it is apparent that such a trial would be ineffective or inappropriate, or has already failed (RCP, 1995). Such circumstances, derived from the literature and by consensus, are given in Tables 3.4 and 3.5.

In the case of children, the PHCT could reasonably do a basic assessment to exclude the circumstances shown in Table 3.6, for which referral to a paediatric urologist or nephrologist, or paediatrician might be appropriate. For those children with straightforward nocturnal enuresis, a referral can be made directly to an existing enuresis or specialist service, where a fuller assessment can be undertaken.

Table 3.4: Circumstances requiring immediate referral to secondary care: urinary incontinence in adults

1. If the diagnosis is unclear
2. The presence of other co-morbid conditions, e.g. recurrent urinary tract infection, neurological conditions, vesico-vaginal fistula, fibroids
3. The presence of marked pelvic prolapse
4. An enlarged prostate if clinically significant
5. An abnormal post-voiding urine volume
6. The presence of microhaematuria without infection
7. After previous continence surgery
8. When a the risk of a therapeutic trial is unacceptable
9. When a therapeutic trial has failed, i.e. when there is no evidence of progress after 2–3 months

Resnick, 1990a; AHCPR, 1992; Walters and Realini, 1992; Bernard, 1994; RCP, 1995.

Table 3.5: Circumstances requiring immediate referral to secondary care: faecal incontinence

1. Suspected inflammatory or malignant bowel disease, e.g. recent diarrhoea, bloody stools
2. Acute faecal impaction not responding to management by the PHCT
3. Neurological disease
4. Suspected sphincter damage (RCP, 1995)
5. When pressing social problems make management in a primary care setting inappropriate
6. Failed therapeutic trial
7. Unresponsive severe constipation in children

Table 3.6: Circumstances requiring immediate referral to secondary care: enuresis in children

1. Daytime wetting and voiding symptoms and abnormal examination
2. Abnormalities on urinalysis and positive midstream urine culture
3. Major bowel disturbance and severe encopresis
4. Nocturnal enuresis in a schoolage child not responding to an alarm/drugs (RCP, 1995)
5. Congenital/neurological causes of urinary incontinence

Clark *et al.*, 1994.

- **The PHCT should have knowledge of available specialist skills to enable appropriate referral.**

Rationale

Referrals for secondary care may be to a variety of health care professionals and will vary according to need and local availability. These may include urologists, gynaecologists, physicians in care of the elderly, paediatricians with a special interest in enuresis, enuresis clinics, neurologists, gastroenterologists and colorectal surgeons. The continence adviser, physiotherapist specialising in continence care and specialist enuresis service may be a part of primary or secondary care depending on local arrangements. There was consensus that information on the specialist services in their area should be available to the PHCT. This should include details of the expertise and interest of individual specialists in order that referral can be to the most suitable person or service. This database could be developed locally by the PHCT or by purchasers who could arrange compilation and distribution.

- **Behavioural techniques may be used successfully by knowledgeable staff to restore or improve continence in some cases. These include:**
  - **bladder re-education programmes;**
  - **conditioning methods;**
  - **pelvic floor re-education;**
  - **biofeedback.**

Bladder re-education programmes

Rationale

These aim to restore urinary continence either by re-educating the bladder to a normal or improved pattern of voiding or by avoiding incontinence episodes through voiding at planned times. Individuals with urgency, urge incontinence and detrusor instability are most likely to benefit, although these techniques have also been used successfully for stress incontinence and with children suffering from daytime wetting. Research studies of these techniques have generally lacked controls and have not involved a long-term follow-up of their efficacy. There are four types of programme:

Bladder training. The time interval between voidings is gradually increased. Intervals may be mandatory or self-adjusted. Individuals must be motivated and able physically and mentally to toilet themselves. It is unclear exactly how this technique works, but it has produced improvements in subjective measures of urinary incontinence, especially in reducing symptoms of urgency and frequency and incontinent episodes in adults (Burgio, 1990; Fantl *et al.*, 1991; Hyland, 1991; O'Brien *et al.*, 1991; Lagro-Janssen, Debruyne, Smits *et al.*, 1992; McDowell *et al.*, 1992; Harrison and Memel, 1994) and children (Meadows, 1990).

Habit training. The time interval between voiding is altered to suit an individual's voiding pattern. It is suitable for individuals with physical or learning disabilities but requires motivated staff or carers (Kennedy, 1992).

Timed voiding. Scheduled toileting to a rigid regime, usually a 2-hourly interval, this technique is often used for institutionalised, debilitated elderly people in whom no individual voiding pattern emerges (Kennedy, 1992).

Prompted voiding. This method utilises a fixed prompting schedule whereby individuals are asked at set times if they wish to void, but it uses a varying voiding schedule. It has been shown to reduce the number of incontinence episodes in institutionalised elderly people (Engel *et al.*, 1990; Schnelle, 1990; Colling *et al.*, 1992; Burgio *et al.*, 1994).

Conditioning methods

Rationale

Enuresis alarms. Around 60–80% children with nocturnal enuresis have been shown to attain dryness within 4 months with treatment using pad and buzzer or body-worn alarms, although success depends on patient selection, education and enthusiasm as well as choice of an appropriate alarm (Gustafson, 1993; van Londen *et al.*, 1993; Butler, 1994; Clark *et al.*, 1994). Such alarms may also be used for adults with nocturnal enuresis (Morgan, 1993) and have been used to aid prompted voiding in the elderly (McCormick *et al.*, 1992).

Minimum standards relating to alarm-based treatments are outlined by ERIC (Morgan, 1993). The supply of and access to alarm equipment is obviously essential to this form of treatment, and the PHCT should try to ensure availability for those who require it.

Dry bed training may also assist alarm therapy. This involves the child rehearsing beforehand the routine that would be involved if woken at night by the alarm (Clark *et al.*, 1994).

Behaviour therapy techniques. These techniques, based on operant conditioning, have been shown to be effective in improving toileting behaviour and continence in individuals with learning difficulties (Roe, 1992b). The use of star charts/rewards to achieve compliance with training tasks for the treatment of enuresis has been shown to be effective in conjunction with other therapies in children (Maizels *et al.*, 1993; Clark *et al.*, 1994).

Pelvic floor re-education

Rationale

The strength and elasticity of the pelvic floor muscles can be restored and improved through pelvic muscle exercises and electrical stimulation.

Pelvic floor exercises. These techniques are generally used for women with stress incontinence and have produced improvements in subjective measures of urinary incontinence, although studies are difficult to compare because of the use of a variety of designs, methods, samples and outcome measure (Cammu *et al.*, 1991; Lagro-Janssen, Debruyne, Smits *et al.*, 1991; Mouritsen *et al.*, 1991; Wells *et al.*, 1991; Dougherty *et al.*, 1993; Elia and Bergman, 1993; Hahn *et al.*, 1993). They have also been used successfully for urge incontinence (Flynn *et al.*, 1994) and with children (Schneider *et al.*, 1994), although these were both small studies.

All females require a digital assessment by a health care professional with the appropriate training in order to check that the woman is contracting the correct muscles (Bump *et al.*, 1991), provide an individualised programme of exercise and evaluate the effectiveness of the exercises (Laycock, 1992). Pelvic floor exercises are most effectively taught by a person with special training.

Vaginal cones. The use of a series of weighed cones as an adjunct to pelvic muscle exercises may help to increase the strength of the muscle contraction and provide proprioceptive feedback (Laycock, 1992). The research evidence of the efficacy of these cones is limited, but the panel felt that this was a low-risk therapy that might be of some use for women who could to some degree contract the correct muscles.

Electrical stimulation. Studies have shown that these techniques can produce some improvement in subjective measures of both stress and urge urinary incontinence but have varied with regard to the actual conditions concerning the electrical stimulation (Fossberg *et al.*, 1990; Esa *et al.*, 1991; Hahn *et al.*, 1991; Meyer *et al.*, 1992; Zöllner-Nielsen and Samuelson, 1992; Caputo *et al.*, 1993; Schiotz, 1994). Varied results have been achieved for faecal incontinence (Barrett, 1992, 1993; Scheuer *et al.*, 1994). There is a need for more standardised research and randomised controlled trials to demonstrate the efficacy of these techniques and optimum approach. Referral is required for both urinary and faecal incontinence sufferers to a physiotherapist with the correct knowledge, expertise and availability of equipment.

Biofeedback

Rationale

Electronic or mechanical instruments have been used to provide feedback to individuals on their physiological activity. The perineometer is one of the simplest of these. The use of biofeedback has improved continence in cases of detrusor instability (O'Donnell and Doyle, 1991). It may assist in pelvic floor rehabilitation (Knight and Laycock, 1994) and has been used for children (Maizels *et al.*, 1993). Biofeedback has also been used with some success to treat anorectal incontinence, although the mode of action remains unclear (Barrett, 1993; Enck, 1993; Bassoti and Whitehead, 1994).

- **Drug therapy:**
  Drugs should generally be used in conjunction with other therapy after contributory factors have been addressed.

Rationale

In almost all cases, the evidence for the use of drug therapy in incontinence is **not** based on adequate research data from randomised controlled trials. Almost all drugs have side-effects. There was therefore consensus amongst the panel that:

1. specific drugs should not be named in the guidelines, since these might rapidly become out of date;
2. other than in exceptional circumstances, drug therapy should not be the first line of treatment for urinary or faecal incontinence or enuresis;
3. drug therapy should generally be used in conjunction with other behavioural therapies, and any contributory factors should have been addressed.

- **Regardless of the drug chosen, the initial dose should be relatively low and titrated to balance side-effects against efficacy.**

Rationale

There was consensus that, since all drugs used have side-effects, dosages should initially be low. Side-effects should be clearly explained to individuals (and/or carers or parents) and doses increased according to need.

- **The PHCT should ensure the education, motivation and support of the individual/carer as this is vital to the success of any treatment.**

Rationale

The motivation and positive participation of the individual, whether adult or child, is a key issue in the success of continence

promotion/restoration strategies. The regular support of motivated staff is also essential to success (Kennedy, 1992; Laycock,
1992; Butler, 1994; Clark *et al.*, 1994). Education of the individual
(and/or carer and parent as appropriate) about the treatment will
also increase compliance and the success of treatment (Roe, 1992b;
Morgan, 1993; Butler, 1994; Clark *et al.*, 1994).

- **The progress of the individual should be reassessed regularly at appropriate time intervals.**

Rationale

The plan of care should incorporate outcome targets and review
dates. Individual progress should then be audited against these
targets in a positive manner by the PHCT (Morgan, 1993; Charter
for Continence, 1995; NHSE, 1995). Regular reviews of progress
will provide opportunities for the motivational support of individuals
by the PHCT.

The periods for review will depend on the particular therapy and
individual need. In general, the panel agreed that 2–3 months was a
reasonable period for a therapeutic trial of behavioural techniques,
regular reviews of progress being made during this time. A decision
should be made about secondary referral after that period. Morgan
(1993) and Clark *et al.* (1994) provide detailed guidelines on follow-up
times for children.

- **All treatments for the promotion and restoration of continence should be undertaken by appropriately trained
  personnel, should conform to preset standards and should
  be subject to audit.**

Rationale

There was consensus that whoever provides treatment for the
restoration of continence should have the appropriate knowledge,
skills and expertise, whether in a primary or secondary care setting.
It was agreed that there was a need for all techniques, including
surgical techniques, to conform to preset standards and be subject to
audit, the results of such audit being available to the PHCT.
Consumer views on treatments should form part of this audit. This
would assist the PHCT in monitoring the effectiveness of treatments
and determining the best care for individuals.

Management of incontinence

- **The restoration of continence should be the aim for all persons. The management of incontinence should occur concurrently with strategies for the restoration of continence or only when such strategies have been shown to fail.**

Rationale

The aim of care for a person suffering from incontinence is return to continence. However, whilst therapy is ongoing or if it is unsuccessful, management of the incontinence in order to achieve social continence is the goal. This can be achieved through the use of a variety of aids, appliances and continence products. No single product suits all individuals, and few aids/appliances have been subjected to adequately controlled trials (Brink, 1990; Cottenden, 1992). Aids/appliances available include containment aids, conduction aids and occlusive devices (Ryan-Wooley, 1987):

Containment aids maybe disposable or reusable:
- body-worn pads/pants;
- underpads used to protect chairs or beds.

Conduction aids:
- male collection appliances (body-worn urinals, penile sheaths);
- female collection appliances;
- catheters (indwelling urethral, suprapubic, clean intermittent catheterisation, including self-catheterisation).

Occlusive devices:
- penile clamps (rarely used).

Other devices:
- pessaries.

The Directory of Aids and Appliances (ACA, 1988) provides information on the pads and appliances available in the United Kingdom. A new directory will be available from the Continence Foundation in 1998.

• **No aid or appliance should be issued without an assessment of need by an appropriately trained health care professional.**

Rationale

The cost to the NHS of providing continence aids and appliances has been estimated to be at least £50 million per annum, with an additional £18 million worth of appliances being provided on prescription in England and Wales (DH, 1991). Individuals may have received pads without a prior assessment by a health care professional, and many of the pads supplied may be inappropriate for the needs of individuals (McKeever, 1990).

An assessment of need should always precede the prescription of any aid or appliance. As soon as possible following initial provision, a thorough assessment should be undertaken of the individual, their incontinence, abilities and disabilities, lifestyle and environment, and that of their carers where appropriate. Selecting the correct size and absorbency of products can aid comfort and security. This can help to enhance the sufferer's quality of life and ability to socialise, and increase the carer's ability to cope (Brink, 1990; Cottenden, 1992; Hellstrom *et al.*, 1993; Philp *et al.*, 1993; Gibb and Wong, 1994).

• **The choice of the individual should be a key consideration in the determination of management approach and selection of aids.**

Rationale

Individual choice and the subjective impression of a product are important (Philp *et al.*, 1992, 1993). Individuals should be provided with information on the range of products available and how to obtain them (Charter for Continence, 1995; NHSE, 1995).

• **The PHCT should ensure that the individual/carer is adequately educated in the correct use of any aid or appliance issued.**

Rationale

Clear instructions, supported if necessary by written information, should be provided to the individual and/or carer on the correct use of all aids and appliances. Feedback should be obtained to check that this has been understood (Cottenden, 1992; Roe, 1992b; Morgan, 1993; Charter for Continence, 1995).

- **All individuals should be regularly reviewed, as their needs may change and/or new management approaches may become available.**

Rationale

There was clear consensus that regular review dates should be set when aids and appliances are issued in order to reassess the individual's requirements. The periods for review will vary according to individual need and the aid/appliance used.

Prevention

- **Opportunities for the prevention of incontinence should be considered by the PHCT.**

Rationale

Whilst there are no research studies to demonstrate which measures will prevent the onset of incontinence, the panel agreed that evidence that effective pelvic floor musculature can improve both urinary and faecal incontinence was sufficient to propose that opportunities for prevention be considered.

The role of midwives and health visitors in advising and teaching pregnant and postnatal women about pelvic floor function and exercise was considered by the panel to be an important factor in continence promotion. However, the panel agreed that it may be rather late to wait until women present at antenatal classes to teach pelvic floor exercises.

Providing individuals with knowledge of the function of the pelvic floor muscles and factors that may affect their function, and encouraging them to exercise these muscles routinely from an early age, may possibly help to reduce problems later in life. This could be provided as an integral part of education about sexual health by school nurses. The effects of such education on pelvic floor function should be evaluated in the future.

Assessment of pelvic floor muscle function should be undertaken by a suitably trained health care professional in all women as part of routine cervical cytology screening. Women could be taught correct pelvic floor exercise technique at this stage.

Improved training for midwives, GPs and obstetricians in the episiotomy technique may help to reduce pelvic floor damage and thus prevent incontinence (RCP, 1995).

The panel also felt that the education of parents about the importance of toileting habits might also reduce problems of faecal incontinence later in life.

Educational issues

- **Each PHCT should have an educational strategy that aims to increase the awareness of all its members of the problems of incontinence.**

Rationale

Since incontinence is a common problem, all members of the PHCT are likely to encounter sufferers during their practice. The amount of time devoted to incontinence and its treatment in the pre-registration education of all health care professionals is relatively little (Brocklehurst, 1990b; Laycock, 1995). There is evidence that the knowledge base of some members of the PHCT regarding the promotion/restoration of continence and the management of incontinence is weak (Briggs and Williams, 1992; Oakshott and Hunt, 1992; Burns *et al.*, 1993; Jolleys and Wilson, 1993). An educational strategy should increase awareness of the nature of the problem of incontinence (including enuresis), its prevalence, the potential for improvement in the majority of cases and the correct use of aids and appliances. This strategy should place emphasis on enhancing the existing skills of the members of the PHCT.

- **There should be opportunities, if necessary, for at least one member of the PHCT to undergo additional training to increase his/her level of knowledge and expertise in relation to incontinence.**

Rationale

There was consensus that the assessment, diagnosis and treatment of incontinence required additional knowledge and expertise. If necessary, arrangements should be made for the relevant member of the PHCT to obtain additional training to enable the individual at least to undertake an assessment, including digital assessment of the pelvic floor muscles, and understand and correctly teach behavioural approaches for the promotion/restoration of the continence. Education need not necessarily be through formal teaching sessions. Continence advisers are best placed to provide multidisciplinary education (Rhodes, 1994), although specialist physiotherapists may be more skilled in pelvic floor assessment and muscle re-education.

Continuous quality improvement

- **There should be nationally agreed standards for the provision of continence care by the PHCT.**

Rationale

Given the number of individual PHCTs, there was consensus within the panel that it would be better for the care of individuals and a better use of resources if standards for the provision of continence services were set nationally and then applied and audited locally.

- **There should be a continuous quality improvement programme for the continence service offered by the PHCT, which should include as a minimum:**
  - **clinical audit using locally agreed outcome measures;**
  - **audit of the educational strategy;**
  - **audit of the knowledge of and commitment of members of the PHCT to the guidelines;**
  - **the appraisal of consumer views.**

Rationale

In order to achieve continuous improvement in the quality of the care given by the PHCT, there was consensus that all aspects of the guidelines and service should be evaluated. This may be achieved by professionally led, locally undertaken clinical audit.

Outcome measures should be locally agreed but may include prevalence rates, referral rates and patterns, numbers of successful treatments, drop-outs from treatment and the provision of aids and appliances. Appropriate record-keeping systems need to be in place to facilitate these audits. The views of individuals and/or their carers who use the continence service should be obtained, possibly through the use of consumer satisfaction surveys.

The level of knowledge and commitment of the PHCT to the guidelines should be audited. The results of all audits should be made known to all members of the PHCT and the conclusions acted upon. Changes should then be made to practice, where warranted, in the light of the audit findings. At an agreed time, repeated audits should be undertaken to assess the extent to which changes in practice have resulted in improvements in care.

- **There should be continuous quality improvement of these guidelines, through regular review and revision as appropriate.**

Rationale

In order to take account of service developments and changes in clinical practice, these guidelines should also be subjected to regular review and revision.

Chapter 4
Systematic review of the literature

Introduction and background

A systematic review of the literature relating to incontinence from 1983 to 1993 had already been undertaken (Williams *et al.*, 1995). A systematic review of the literature for urinary and faecal incontinence for the years 1990 to 1994 was therefore undertaken for these consensus guidelines.

The methods used for the literature search and review are presented, including the limitations of the review. This literature review aims to evaluate the research base of care provided by the PHCT for the promotion and management of continence. Areas of consensus within the literature are highlighted and summarised.

The literature on urinary incontinence is systematically reviewed in relation to the prevalence, incidence, burden of incontinence, assessment, promotion and management of continence. The literature on faecal incontinence is briefly discussed, and the educational and audit issues related to the promotion of continence are outlined.

Literature search and review methodology

A search was undertaken of relevant literature published between January 1990 and November 1994. The CD-Rom database MEDLINE on Dialog software was searched using the following medical subject headings:

INCONTINENCE-FECAL
INCONTINENCE-URINARY

INCONTINENCE-STRESS
INCONTINENCE-PADS

and including all relevant subheadings. The search was modified to include only publications in English and those referring to HUMANS. The CD-Rom CINAHL database was also searched using Silverplatter software and the search term '*INCONTINENCE*'. In addition, relevant current journals held in the John Rylands Library at the University of Manchester were searched manually in November 1994, since these would not yet have been indexed on MEDLINE. Relevant articles retrieved through a hand search of the journal *Neurourology and Urodynamics* were acquired through personal communication with Dr B. Roe, since this journal only appeared on MEDLINE from 1994.

Inclusion criteria

Publications were considered eligible for inclusion if they were:

• published between January 1990 and November 1994;
• published in English;
• original research or reviews of the literature;
• published before January 1990 but identified as key papers through repeated citations by later authors;
• related directly or indirectly to the promotion of continence and management of incontinence by the PHCT.

Exclusion criteria

Because of the time constraints of the project and inherent weaknesses in the studies, the following publications were excluded:

• anecdotal reports;
• case studies;
• uncontrolled trials of treatments;
• studies dealing with topics outside the remit of the PHCT, e.g. those relating to the surgical management of incontinence.

Clinical questions

Following the model adopted by Cullum (1994) for reviewing the literature on leg ulcers, a series of clinical questions was posed in order to direct the literature review. It was assumed that publications addressing the following clinical questions would be most relevant to the review and therefore be included:

1. What is incontinence (urinary and faecal)?
2. What is the prevalence and incidence of incontinence (urinary and faecal)?
3. What factors may lead to the development of incontinence and exacerbate the problem?
4. What are the costs of incontinence to both the patient and in financial terms?
5. How should incontinence be assessed?
6. How should continence be promoted by the PHCT?
7. How should incontinence be managed by the PHCT?
8. When and how should referral to other professionals be undertaken?
9. How can the outcomes of the promotion and management of continence be audited?
10. How can professionals, patients and the public be educated about incontinence?

Questions remaining unanswered by the literature would, as Cullum (1994) has pointed out, identify and guide areas for further research.

Publications included in the review were categorised according to the clinical questions that they addressed. Literature included in the review included literature reviews and original research. Further questions were then asked of these publications in order to determine the quality of the evidence presented.

Literature reviews

Reviews of previous research were considered relevant to this study, especially since time prevented a search of literature earlier than 1990. Thorough reviews of the research literature therefore had the potential to provide a useful summary of the state of the art to that time. Judgements were made of the quality of such reviews before their inclusion by the use of questions modified from Mulrow (1987):

- Was the review systematic and was the methodology explained?
- Was it comprehensive?
- Was it critical?
- What was the purpose of the review?
- Was the analysis of research data qualitative or quantitative?
- Were conclusions drawn identifying further research?

Research studies

The following questions, modified from those used by Williams and Roe (1994), were posed of published empirical studies, enabling a judgement to be made on the quality of the report. If a publication failed to meet these requirements, it was not included in the review since insufficient data would be present on which to proceed in determining the quality of the actual study:

- Was the study clear, concise and relevant?
- Were the objectives of the study clearly stated?
- Were the research design and methods and sampling techniques clearly described?
- Were the results comprehensively reported?
- Were recommendations made in the conclusions clear and did they relate to the study's stated objectives?

The quality of the study was then evaluated by considering:

1. the appropriateness of the design and methodology to the aims of the study;
2. possible threats to the internal and external validity of the study;
3. evidence used to support the conclusions drawn.

Additional literature

Copies of relevant Department of Health policy documents were obtained. Examples of existing guidelines and useful sources on the promotion and management of continence were also retrieved from relevant organisations. These have been included in the literature review where appropriate and are summarised in Appendix I.

Limitations

The review was limited by several factors. The search was limited to only those publications indexed on MEDLINE and CINAHL databases, with the exception of *Neurourology and Urodynamics* and publications retrieved through the hand search of current journals. It focuses only on the literature from 1990, other than earlier key papers. It is also limited by the time available for its completion, which prevented some publications being acquired through interlibrary loans.

Use of the chosen search terms did not retrieve literature relating to enuresis, encopresis or prostatism, which are indexed using other medical subject headings. Time did not permit a search and thorough review of this literature. However, the CD-Rom database MEDLINE on Dialog software was searched using the medical subject heading '*ENURESIS*' for literature published from January 1990 to November 1994. This was reviewed briefly, and relevant literature is included in this review.

Nonetheless, this forms a systematic review of the available literature pertaining to the promotion and management of continence by the PHCT.

Definition of incontinence

A standardised definition of urinary incontinence was produced by a committee of the International Continence Society (ICS) (Andersen *et al.*, 1988, p.17):

> urinary incontinence is the involuntary loss of urine which is objectively demonstrable and a social or hygienic problem.

Urinary incontinence can denote a symptom–when the patient complains of involuntary loss of urine; a sign–the objective demonstration of that urine loss; and a condition–when the urine loss is demonstrated urodynamically (Andersen *et al.*, 1988).

Despite the availability of this standardised definition, many authors continue to use alternatives, evidenced by the fact that in over 20 studies published since 1990 of the prevalence of urinary incontinence (Table 4.1) below, only three authors (Borrie and Davidson, 1992; Molander, 1993; North, 1994) have used the ICS definition. Of these, only Borrie and Davidson (1992) and Molander (1993) demonstrated urine loss objectively. Other authors have defined urinary incontinence themselves (Burgio *et al.*, 1991; Cutler *et al.*, 1992; Rekers *et al.*, 1992), often including a time element such as 'the occurrence of incontinence within the past two months' in order to narrow the focus of the study (Ju *et al.*, 1991; O'Brien *et al.*, 1991; Lagace *et al.*, 1993).

The following standardised definition for enuresis in children is endorsed by ERIC and has been adopted for this review (Forsythe and Butler, 1989, p. 879).

> the involuntary discharge of urine by day or night or both, in a child aged five years or older, in the absence of congenital or acquired defects of the nervous system or urinary tract.

There is no equivalent standardised definition for faecal incontinence, although authors have offered their own definitions, e.g. 'the involuntary expulsion of faeces at least once per week in the previous month' (Barrett *et al.*, 1990) and 'the involuntary passage of faeces' (Caputo and Benson, 1992).

Roe and Williams (1994, p. 1) have adapted the ICS definition to encompass both urinary and faecal incontinence as follows:

> A condition where involuntary loss of urine [or faeces] is a social or hygienic problem and is objectively demonstrable.

Since the inclusion of faecal incontinence in this way does not alter the intent of the ICS definition, it is recommended that this definition be accepted for the purpose of this review.

The adoption by researchers and authors of various definitions of incontinence creates difficulties in comparing the results of studies. It is therefore recommended that researchers should, whenever possible, utilise the standardised definitions in order to facilitate comparisons of data and meta-analysis.

Prevalence of urinary incontinence

Following a systematic review of studies of the prevalence of urinary incontinence until 1990, Mohide (1992) concluded that these yielded varying results depending on the definitions of incontinence, samples, methods of data collection and settings used, and that comparisons of studies were not possible. A similar review of published studies of prevalence of urinary incontinence in community settings since 1990, as shown in Table 4.1, demonstrates that this situation has not changed.

Studies have continued to use a variety of definitions of incontinence. Some definitions used and questions asked were very broad, e.g. 'Have you ever leaked even a small amount of urine involuntarily?' (Burgio *et al.*, 1991). Such studies produced prevalence rates of between 52% and 60% in women (Burgio *et al.*, 1991; Cutler *et al.*, 1992; Harrison and Memel, 1994), suggesting that one in every two women has at some time experienced involuntary urine loss. This does not measure, though, the degree to which this is a problem for women.

The use of the standardised ICS definition of urinary incontinence would enhance studies of prevalence and enable comparisons of data to be made. However, the use of the ICS definition of urinary incontinence in prevalence studies should include an objective demonstration of urinary incontinence and confirmation that the urinary incontinence is a social or hygienic problem to the individual. Only three studies used this definition, of which only Molander (1993) verified self-reporting of urinary incontinence by objective demonstration. North (1994) did not objectively demonstrate urinary incontinence nor attempt to identify it as a social or hygienic problem to the individuals concerned.

Use of the ICS definition would exclude those people whose urinary incontinence is not demonstrable objectively, which was 5.7% of women who reported urinary incontinence in Molander's (1993) study. It may also reduce the prevalence rates by only including those individuals who perceive urinary incontinence to be a problem and may exclude some of the large numbers (50–60%) of women in the studies by Burgio et al. (1991) and Cutler et al. (1992) who reported experiencing loss of urine involuntarily at some point in their lives. However, Fultz and Herzog (1993) note that urinary incontinence is a condition that can be gradual, intermittent and longstanding, and that individuals may consequently have adjusted their lifestyles to an extent that urinary incontinence is no longer immediately perceived by them to be a problem but an acceptable part of life. Such individuals would be excluded by the ICS definition yet may suffer severe incontinence.

The very nature of incontinence as a social or hygienic problem mitigates against accurate measurement of its prevalence since individuals are likely to feel embarrassed or ashamed and not wish to admit to the problem (Herzog and Fultz, 1990; Mohide, 1992).

Samples, settings and methods have also varied and not all methods used are adequately described, so comparisons cannot be made between studies. Only one study (Fonda, 1990) stated that it had measured dependent continence, i.e. cases where, without physical help or regular toileting, individuals would have been incontinent. Mohide (1992) points out the need for studies to clarify whether catheterised individuals are included in studies of the prevalence of urinary incontinence since institutional studies fail to include such people.

Only four studies focused specifically on prevalence in children (Hellstrom et al., 1990b; Devlin, 1991; Bloom et al., 1993; Swithinbank et al., 1994) and the majority related to urinary incontinence in women. Studies of incontinence in men may be related more specifically to symptoms of disorders of the prostate, and these may not have been retrieved through this literature search.

'Recognised' incontinence was only studied by McKeever (1990), who found the prevalence of incontinence, as shown by those known to the health authority, to be very low (0.47%), but she did not include those people known only to social services or GPs.

Table 4.1: Summary of studies of prevalence of urinary incontinence published since 1990

Study	Sample	Population and setting	Definition	Data source	Data collection	Prevalence	Comments
Hellstrom *et al.* (1990a)	85-year-old men and women $N = 954$	Gothenburg, Sweden. All men and women aged 85 in 1986 $N = 1502$	'The occurrence of involuntary urinary leakage – confirmed by pad test'	Subjects	Face-to-face interviews and medical examination by urotherapist. Response rate 64.8%	37.2% 43% female 24% male	Included both institutionalised and non-institutionalised persons. Significantly more female non-respondents, lived at home than respondents
Lagro-Janssen *et al.* (1990)	Random sample of women aged 50–65 $N = 1442$	75 General practices in eastern part of The Netherlands	Involuntary loss of urine more than twice per month	Subjects	Interviewed at home by trained interviewers. Response rate 60%	22.5%	Not clear whether interviewers were health professionals

Study	Setting/population	Definition	Source	Method	Results	Comments
McKeever (1990)	A single district health authority in Great Britain that did not have a continence adviser at the time. Population served not given. Recognised incontinence, i.e. all those living in the community and receiving assistance from the health authority as a direct result of incontinence. Those receiving care from GPs and having no contact with the authority were excluded, as were those dealing only with social services $N = 847$	'Assumed that by receiving these services people were incontinent, therefore no definition of incontinence was included as a criterion for selection'	Community nurses and health visitors, registers of those receiving incontinence products	Community staff visiting incontinent people on a regular basis given a questionnaire. Not clear how it was determined who to send it to. No details of follow-up procedures or response rates. Registers recording details of those people receiving incontinence products were used; a 10% random sample of these people was interviewed later	Recognised incontinence 0.47%	Sample does not include those being treated by GPs or known only to social services. Details of procedures used to identify relevant people are not clear
Simeonova and Bengtsson (1990)	Gothenburg, Sweden. Women aged 18 and over visiting health centre $N = 550$	'Involuntary voiding of urine'	Subjects	Questionnaire handed to subjects at health centre. Response rate 82%	44%	

(contd)

Table 4.1: (contd)

Study	Sample	Population and setting	Definition	Data source	Data collection	Prevalence	Comments
Burgio et al. (1991)	Women aged 42–50 recruited as part of 'Healthy women study' N = 541	Population of women with driver's licence in selected zip codes of Pittsburgh, USA N = 2405; those who fulfilled criteria for inclusion = 901	'Have you ever leaked even a small amount of urine involuntarily?'	Subjects	Initial selection via telephone interview – response rate 60%. Face-to-face interviews with nurse at clinic	58.4%	(30.7% reported incontinence at lease once per month)
Ju et al. (1991)	Men and women aged 65 or over N = 919	Residents aged 65 or over on a public housing estate in Singapore N = 1143	Leakage of urine on at lease two occasions in the past month	Subjects	Interviewed in homes by medical students. Response rate 80.4%	4.6% 4.4% male 4.8% female	
O'Brien et al. (1991)	Random sample adults aged 35 and over N = 7300	Adults aged 35 and over on two general practice lists in Somerset, UK (one urban, one rural) N = 10300	Regular incontinence — two or more leaks of urine in any one month	Subjects	Postal questionnaire; reminders sent after 4 weeks. Response rate 79%. Those reporting regular incontinence were followed up either by phone or in person and their responses validated	4.4% male 16.4% female	

| Cutler et al. (1992) | (a) Premenopausal women who were part of a study on the menopause in 1979. Mean age 48.67. $N = 57$

(b) Women participating in an 'executive level' wellness evaluation. $N = 137$

Total $N = 194$ | (a) Women participating in the Stanford Menopause study, USA; details of population not given

(b) Healthy women who participated in the Athena Wellness Program, Pennsylvania, USA, undergoing the 2½ hour $300 wellness evaluation. Due to the cost of the examination, women were either management executive level and/or of high socio-economic status | (a) 'Loss of urine sometimes occurs involuntarily. Does this ever happen to you?'

(b) 'Do you have trouble with involuntary urine loss?' Further questions were then asked about severity, etc. | (a) and (b) Subjects | (a) Face-to-face interview with the researcher at Stanford

(b) Questionnaire completed in private at the clinic during the wellness evaluation. Pelvic muscle testing provided as part of the evaluation for some participants Response rate 98% | (a) 60%

(b) 52% | Both samples small. Samples neither random nor representative of general public. Definitions of incontinence very broad |

(contd)

Table 4.1: (contd)

Study	Sample	Population and setting	Definition	Data source	Data collection	Prevalence	Comments
Kok *et al.* (1992)	Stratified random sample of community-residing women aged 60 and over (excluding those in institutions) $N = 1049$	Female residents of municipality of Amstelveen, The Netherlands, aged 60 and over on 31/12/1988 $N = 8967$	Involuntary loss of urine at least twice a week, irrespective of amount of urine lost	Subjects	Postal questionnaire; reminder sent 3 weeks later. Response rate 69%	23.5%	Study says that questionnaires were anonymous so no additional information available from non-respondents, yet it states that reminders were sent
Rekers *et al.* (1992)	Stratified sample of women aged between 35 and 80 years; two-thirds of those selected were between 45 and 64 years old $N = 1299$	Zoetermeer, The Netherlands	Involuntary loss or urine	Subjects	Postal questionnaire; reminders sent after 2 and 4 months. Response rate 67.7%. Included questions on consequences of incontinence	26.5%	

Study	Sample	Setting	Definition/Question	Respondents	Method	Prevalence	Non-response
Brocklehurst (1993)	Random sample of adults aged 30 years or over living at home $N = 4007$	178 constituency sampling points in Great Britain	'Have you ever suffered from any of these health problems – bladder problems e.g. leaking, wet pants, damp pants'	Subjects	Face-to-face interviews in the home using standardised format by market researchers. No response rate given	14.0% female 6.6% male	No response rate given
Lagace et al. (1993)	All men and women aged 20 years and older who visited family physicians/offices for any reason during an 11 week period (July–Sept 1990) $N = 2830$	Five family practice offices in UPRNet, Upper Peninsula, Michigan, USA Population = 20 779 Number of eligible patients = 3638	'Current urinary incontinence' was defined as any degree of incontinence in the past 12 months	Subjects. Carers were able to complete answers for 'mentally retarded adults'	Anonymous questionnaire completed in the practice offices and left in a box. Question also asked about severity and consequences of incontinence. Responses from women whose incontinence occurred only while pregnant were excluded. Response rate = 77.8%	33% 11% male 43% female	No details on non-respondents

(contd)

Table 4.1: (contd)

Study	Sample	Population and setting	Definition	Data source	Data collection	Prevalence	Comments
Molander (1993)	Stratified random sample of women aged 46–85 years $N = 7459$	Female population aged 46–86 years in Gothenburg, Sweden $N = 91044$	ICS definition: a condition in which the involuntary loss of urine is a social and hygienic problem and is objectively demonstrable	Subjects	Postal questionnaire; follow-up letter sent after 12 weeks. Response rate 74.6%. Subsample ($N = 350$) of women complaining of incontinence were assessed at continence clinic and incontinence demonstrated objectively using 48-hour pad test, micturition lists and a cough provocation test	12.1–25%, increasing in linear fashion with age	No significant differences between respondents and non-respondents regarding place of residence, e.g. own home, institution. No other apparent differences. Urinary incontinence not objectively demonstrable in 20 of the 350 women (5.7%)
Sandvik et al. (1993b)	All women aged 20 years and over $N = 182$	Women aged 20 years and over in rural community of Rissa, Norway $N = 2366$	Not specifically defined; questions were asked about duration, frequency and amount of leakage and its impact	Subjects	Postal questionnaire; reminder sent after 1 month. Included a severity index. Response rate 77%	29.4%	Severity index was validated using pad weighing tests

Harrison and Memel (1994)	Random sample (10%) of women aged 20 years or older and not pregnant $N = 384$	One general practice in Bristol, UK $N = 11\ 873$	Not specifically defined. Patient asked about presence of urine leakage, frequency of leakage episodes and whether they leaked urine when they coughed, laughed or exercised	Subjects	Postal questionnaire No follow-up procedures reported. Response rate 82.6%	53.2%
North (1994)	Random stratified sample of women aged between 16 and 85 $N = 1194$	Six general practices in Huddersfield Health Authority, UK. Population 211 414	ICS definition: a condition in which the involuntary loss of urine is a social and hygienic problem and is objectively demonstrable	Subjects. Carers in 69 cases	Postal questionnaire; no details of reminders. Response rate 58.7%. Sufferers invited to attend clinic	20.60% (undefined problem)

North (1994) comments: Although report claimed to use ICS definition, questions asked did not focus on social and hygienic aspects, nor was incontinence objectively demonstrable

(contd)

Table 4.1: (contd)

Study	Sample	Population and setting	Definition	Data source	Data collection	Prevalence	Comments
Wolfs *et al.* (1994)	All male patients aged 55 or older $N = 2734$	10 general practices in Maastricht, The Netherlands (population 115 000)	No definition given: symptom inventory used	Subject	Postal questionnaire comprising symptom inventory. Two written follow-up reminders sent. Response rate 64.3%. Further clarification of replies achieved when necessary by phone interview or reference to medical records	10.5%	7.2% did not answer the question on incontinence 48.8% reported symptoms of dribbling

Studies in Institutional Settings

Study	Sample	Population and setting	Definition	Data source	Data collection	Prevalence	Comments
Fonda (1990)	All residents $N = 1659$	10 geriatric short-stay assessment/ rehabilitation services and long-stay nursing homes in Victoria, Australia	Unkown: did include dependent continence, i.e. 'being dry of urine only as a result of being reminded or physically assisted'	Nursing home staff	One-day census. Data collected by nursing staff reports	Short-stay residents: 31% incontinent 26% dependent continent. Nursing home residents: 66% incontinent 11% dependent continent	Details of methodology brief

Study	Sample	Definition	Respondents	Method	Prevalence	Comments
Borrie and Davidson (1992)	All inpatients who met required criteria. Mean age 73 years $N = 457$. Long-term care hospital, Ontario, Canada	ICS definition: the involuntary loss of urine which is a social and hygienic problem and is objectively demonstrable	Nursing staff	Questionnaire completed by staff; nurses, reports verified by hospital records Response rate 92%	62%	Not clear how social/hygienic problem was defined for staff. Objective demonstration of urinary incontinence by nurses' observation
Ouslander et al. (1993)	All newly admitted residents aged 65 over $N = 430$. Eight proprietary nursing homes in Maryland, USA	Daytime incontinence: not defined	Nursing home staff	Nurses' aides reports of continence status; details not given	39%	Methodology not fully reported
Studies of Prevalence in Children						
Hellstrom et al. (1990b)	7-year-old school entrants $N = 3556$. Gothenburg, Sweden	Unknown	Parents/ guardians	Postal questionnaire on micturition habits supplemented by phone interviews. Response rate ?	Nocturnal enuresis 7.0% boys 2.8% girls. Nocturnal incontinence and daytime wetting 2.0% boys 2.3% girls	No response rate given

(contd)

Table 4.1: (contd)

Study	Sample	Population and setting	Definition	Data source	Data collection	Prevalence	Comments
Devlin (1991)	Cluster sample of schoolchildren aged 4–14 years $N = 1806$	Six primary schools in Co. Kildare, Ireland	Enuresis defined as 'involuntary urination during sleep, occurring at least once a month in children over 4 years of age'	Parents/ guardians	Self-administered questionnaire given to parents/guardians. Response rate 98%	Nocturnal enuresis 13% boys 15% girls 12%	Non-respondents did not differ from respondents
Bloom et al. (1993)	Opportunity sample of children $N = 1806$	Michigan, USA	Daytime wetting and nocturnal enuresis not defined	Parents/ guardians	Questionnaires and structured interview	Diurnal enuresis – 10% Nocturnal enuresis – 18%	
Swithinbank et al. (1994)	Children starting year 7 (11–12 years) secondary school in 1992 $N = 1176$ (115 boys, 665 girls)	16 out of 19 secondary schools in Southmead area of Bristol, UK	Nocturnal enuresis: 'bedwetting at least once every 3 months'. Diurnal enuresis: 'wetting of pants with some regularity'	Subjects	Self-administered questionnaire give to children. Questionnaire related to urinary symptoms and incontinence. Response rate 59.2%	Nocturnal enuresis 6.2% boys 3.5% girls. Diurnal enuresis 7.2% boys 16.6% girls	Part of longit-udinal study of urinary symptoms in secondary schoolchildren

Pre-1990 study most commonly cited

Thomas et al. (1980)	(a) Recognised incontinence all those aged 15 and over known to health or social services N = 1944 (b) Unrecognised incontinence all patients aged 5 and over	London Boroughs and Health Districts of Brent and Harrow, UK N = 359 000 12 general practices in five districts of England	Regular incontinence – involuntary leakage of urine in inappropriate places or at inappropriate times – twice or more a month regardless of the quantity of urine lost. Incontinence occurring less than twice a month = occasional	(a) Health and social service agencies (b) Subjects and parents/ guardians of those aged 5–15	(a) No details of standard questionnaire, no follow-up procedures reported. No response rate (b) Postal questionnaire, two reminders sent after 3 weeks. Response rate 87%	(a) Less than 1% aged 15–64, 2% aged over 65 (b) 16% 15–64 years 22% over 65 years	Few details given on methodology used by health and social service agencies

Although direct comparisons and a meta-analysis of prevalence studies cannot be made owing to the differences outlined, from the evidence of this review and those of Mohide (1992) and Williams and Roe (1994), it is apparent that urinary incontinence is a very common problem affecting all ages.

Prevalence rates of between 1.6% and 6.6% have been found for men aged over 15 years (Thomas et al., 1980; O'Brien et al., 1991; Brocklehurst, 1993), with a rise to 6.9–10.5% for men aged over 55 years (Thomas et al., 1980; Wolfs et al., 1994).

Studies of prevalence have shown that urinary incontinence is more common in women, being reported by 8.6% of women aged 16–64 years (Thomas et al., 1980) and objectively demonstrated in 12.1–25% of women aged 46–85 years, increasing in linear fashion with age (Molander, 1993). In addition, 1% of adults are reported to have nocturnal enuresis (Thomas et al., 1980; O'Brien et al., 1991; Brocklehurst, 1993; Molander, 1993).

Nocturnal enuresis in children is reported in 15% of children aged 5 years (Clark et al., 1994) and 7% of boys and 3% of girls aged 7 years (Hellstrom et al., 1990b). Day- and night-time wetting occurs in 2 –10% of schoolchildren (Hellstrom et al., 1990b; Bloom et al., 1993). However, 15–16% of children who bedwet experience spontaneous remission each year (Clark et al., 1994).

The prevalence in elderly people in institutions was found to be between 31% and 60% depending on the type of residential accommodation (Fonda, 1990; Borrie and Davidson, 1992; Ouslander, 1993).

Despite the number of new prevalence studies, some of which utilised stringent methods and only included urinary incontinence demonstrated objectively (Molander, 1993), none has been as large as that undertaken by Thomas et al. (1980) in the United Kingdom. This therefore continues to be the study most often quoted by authors on urinary incontinence, even though the data collection methodology was not clearly reported and the study is now 18 years old.

Most of the prevalence rates given in the studies since 1990 are higher than those found by Thomas et al. (1980), which are included in Table 4.1 above for information. It would be useful to know whether this is due to the differences in methodology, setting, definition of urinary incontinence and sample used, or whether it in any way reflects the increasing public awareness about incontinence over the past 18 years. Such increasing awareness may have led to a reduction in the stigma attached to the condition, thereby enabling individuals to be more open about the problem. The MORI poll on incontinence was undertaken more recently in the United Kingdom (Brocklehurst, 1993) but was still of a limited sample size and used a very broad definition of incontinence. Although 4007 people were interviewed by market researchers, no data are given on the response rate.

There are, therefore, several recent prevalence studies available, only a few of which have been undertaken in the United Kingdom (McKeever, 1990; O'Brien et al., 1991; Brocklehurst, 1993; Harrison and Memel, 1994; North, 1994). Consequently, there seems little need for further small prevalence studies. None of the recent studies was as large as that by Thomas et al. (1980). There may be a need for a study of the scale undertaken by Thomas et al. in the United Kingdom in order to provide more recent figures on recognised and unrecognised incontinence in this country. Research undertaken for the Department of Health as part of the project evaluating health interventions by continence advisory services and PHCTs on patient outcomes related to incontinence will provide a more recent prevalence on the basis of a large postal survey (Roe, 1995, personal communication). However, it is evident from this review, and seems generally to be accepted, that incontinence is a common problem affecting both sexes across the whole age spectrum, its prevalence being greatest in women and elderly people. Resources would be utilised more effectively, therefore, in dealing with the problem than measuring its size.

Incidence of urinary incontinence

The incidence of urinary incontinence has not been studied as fully as its prevalence (Herzog and Fultz, 1990). Three incidence studies published since 1990 were found, none of which arose from within the United Kingdom.

Herzog, Diokno et al. (1990) interviewed a probability sample of 1956 non-institutionalised people aged 60 and over in their own homes in Michigan, at annual intervals. One-year incidence rates were approximately 20% for women and 10% for men. Remission rates for previously incontinent persons were 12% for women and 30% for men.

In a follow-up of 206 women aged 42–50 years involved in the prevalence study reported in Table 4.1 above, Burgio et al. (1991) found that, over 3 years, 8% developed a problem of at least monthly leakage of urine.

The incidence of urinary incontinence in institutionalised individuals was studied by Ouslander et al. (1993) by assessing daytime incontinence in 430 people aged 65 and over on admission to eight nursing homes and thereafter at periods of 2 months and 1 year. Incidence was found to be greater in men than women at both 2 months and 1 year (21% females, 51% males, and 16% females, 46% males respectively). Women's incontinence was more likely to resolve than men's, since 23% of women's urinary incontinence had resolved after 1 year compared with 14% of men's.

The paucity of incidence studies makes it difficult to draw many conclusions from the data, and in the few studies that exist, the settings, methods and samples vary considerably, so comparisons are not possible. Ouslander *et al.* (1993) were able to show that the development of urinary incontinence was associated with male sex, a diagnosis of dementia, immobility and faecal incontinence. This was, however, with a sample of elderly institutionalised people and is therefore not representative of the general public. Further incidence studies may be of use, especially in a United Kingdom setting. These may help to highlight factors involved in the development of urinary incontinence, or indeed its remission, and therefore be of use in the prevention of incontinence.

The burden of urinary incontinence

Health care costs

Published empirical studies of the health care costs in the United Kingdom could not be found. Incontinence is not always diagnosed as a condition, so even where it has been reported to a doctor, it may not be recorded in a way that is retrievable for audit. It is, therefore, difficult to measure actual costs.

Hu (1990) identified the direct costs of incontinence as those incurred by the health care system and included the costs of assessment, diagnosis, rehabilitation and aids if finally necessary. The cost consequences were also identified, including the treatment of skin irritation, urinary tract infection and long-stay care, since incontinence has been found to be one of the factors predisposing to institutionalisation (Ouslander, Zarit *et al.*, 1990; O'Donnell *et al.*, 1992). The indirect costs were described by Hu (1990) as the time and money spent by the individuals themselves or their carers.

In estimating the direct health care costs for urinary incontinence in the USA, Hu concluded that over $10 billion was spent in 1987; $7 billion in the community and $3 in institutions.

Financial data on the costs of incontinence in the United Kingdom given by the Department of Health (1991) were provided by the

Association for Continence Advice. Details of the methodology used for the calculations are not given, nor are references to the sources. Since no other published figures were found, these are included as estimates of costs, although they are now several years out of date.

Fifty million pounds per annum was spent directly on pads and appliances, an additional £18 million-worth of appliances being provided on prescription in England and Wales (DH, 1991). These figures do not include all aspects as calculated in the figures by Hu (1990) and rely solely on the expense of the provision of aids and appliances. If all direct costs were calculated, including assessment, diagnosis and treatment, these figures would be far higher. The AHCPR consensus guidelines concluded that significant cost savings could be made if the clinical guidelines on urinary incontinence were to be implemented, although this has yet to be tested empirically (AHCPR, 1992).

It is worth noting, however, that the implementation of guidelines might initially increase expenditure as public awareness is raised, individuals realise the benefits of the guidelines and access the health care system. As the health care costs would include assessment, diagnosis and treatment, increased awareness of professionals might also lead to increased referrals.

There is a need for up-to-date data on the health care costs of incontinence in the United Kingdom. In order to achieve this, there is a need for improved record-keeping by health professionals in relation to incontinence, such that patients complaining of the symptom, and not only those who have a diagnosis of a condition, are identifiable. A feasibility study to measure the economic costs of incontinence within a number of United Kingdom health authorities and Trusts has been undertaken by the Centre for Health Economics and Social Policy Research Unit, University of York, on behalf of the Department of Health. This research is ongoing.

Costs to the patient/carer–financial

Details of the financial costs to the sufferer of incontinence are again difficult to calculate. Indications can be retrieved, however, from studies that have asked sufferers about coping strategies. In a survey of 10 427 people responding to an advertisement for an incontinence self-help group in America, Jeter and Wagner (1990) found that 6.6% were spending more than $30 per month on incontinence and 83% were spending less than $15 per month. Comparable figures for the United Kingdom are not available, but of the 19% of incontinence sufferers using pads in a study in this country by O'Brien *et al.* (1991), 95% had provided these themselves.

Most studies on the effects of incontinence for the individual have shown that women manage their incontinence using sanitary towels and pads rather than specific incontinence pads (Jeter and Wagner, 1990; O'Brien *et al.*, 1991; Rekers *et al.*, 1992; Sandvik *et al.*, 1993). Indeed, some people were using paper towels (Jeter and Wagner, 1990), while others used babies' nappies (Sandvik *et al.*, 1993). No figures are available for the costs of the provision of sanitary products by these people, although in the study by Rekers *et al.* (1992), 125 out of 344 female incontinence sufferers regularly used two sanitary towels a day to manage their condition.

Other costs identified by sufferers include the extra laundry, a problem identified by 68% of women (Sandvik *et al.*, 1993) and 52% of men (Hunskaar and Sandvik, 1993).

These studies all focused on urinary incontinence. The costs involved in faecal or double incontinence would inevitably be higher. Hu (1990) also considers the costs of time off work for the sufferer, either directly because of the problem or for investigations and medical appointments.

Overall, whilst actual details are hard to provide, it can be concluded that individuals and their carers are incurring significant costs as they attempt to manage the incontinence themselves.

Costs to the patient/carer–personal

In reviewing the psychosocial effects of incontinence, Wyman *et al.* (1990) note that, as in the case of prevalence studies, there are no common definitions used and little common methodology. Studies reviewed since 1990 continue to fall into the three categories described by Wyman *et al.*:

1. *Epidemiological studies*, in which data on effects were recorded as part of prevalence studies (Nygaard *et al.*, 1990; O'Brien *et al.*, 1991; Goldstein *et al.*, 1992; Lam *et al.*, 1992; Rekers *et al.*, 1992; Brocklehurst, 1993; Herzog *et al.*, 1994; Reymert and Hunskaar, 1994).
2. *Clinical studies*, whereby sufferers are contacted, for example through advertisements for aids or by attending e.g. urodynamic clinics, and are then surveyed (Jeter and Wagner, 1990; Ouslander and Abelson, 1990; Walters *et al.*, 1990; Macaulay *et al.*, 1991; Vinsnes and Hunskaar, 1991; Lagro-Janssen, Smits *et al.*, 1992;

Clark and Romm, 1993; Grimby *et al.*, 1993; Hunskaar and Sandvik, 1993; Sandvik *et al.*, 1993; Vierhout and Gianotten, 1993).

3. *Ethnographic studies*, in which small samples have been used, usually involving semistructured interviews and attempting to study the experiences of the sufferers in greater depth (Dowd, 1991; Klemm and Creason, 1991; Thomas and Morse, 1991; Ashworth and Hagan, 1993; Birgersson *et al.*, 1993; Skoner and Haylor, 1993).

Incontinence itself does not contribute to or predict mortality (Herzog *et al.*, 1994). For some sufferers, incontinence does not affect their lives; indeed, of 146 women presenting to their doctor with incontinence, 23 declined to take part in a study of the effects as it 'was not a problem', and of those who participated, only 7% said that it was an extreme inconvenience (Lagro-Janssen, Smits *et al.*, 1992). Twenty-three per cent of those with urinary incontinence felt no effect on their lifestyle (Brocklehurst, 1993), and 24% of men responding to an advertisement for aids felt their urinary incontinence to be a negligible problem (Hunskaar and Sandvik, 1993).

However, the majority of sufferers do report the negative effects and personal costs of their condition, often in terms of distress, embarrassment and inconvenience (Ouslander and Abelson, 1990; Lagro-Janssen, Smits *et al.*, 1992; Brocklehurst, 1993). Distress was greater in sufferers of urge incontinence than stress incontinence (Vinsnes and Hunskaar, 1991; Grimby *et al.*, 1993; Sandvik *et al.*, 1993) and in younger sufferers (Hunskaar and Vinsnes, 1991; Hunskaar and Sandvik, 1993), and was related to the amount of urine lost rather than the frequency of incontinence (Ouslander and Abelson, 1990; Lagro-Janssen, Smits *et al.*, 1992). Macaulay *et al.* (1991), undertaking psychiatric assessments of women attending a urodynamic clinic, found one-quarter of sufferers of urinary incontinence to be as depressed, anxious and phobic as psychiatric patients.

Changes and restrictions to patterns of social activity have been reported as a result of urinary incontinence, including avoiding exercise and lifting and going out less (Nygaard *et al.*, 1990; Thomas and Morse, 1991; Lagro-Janssen, Smits *et al.*, 1992; Brocklehurst, 1993). In comparing 120 female sufferers of incontinence with a non-suffering control group, Grimby *et al.* (1993) found incontinence sufferers to be socially more isolated.

The effects of incontinence on sexual activity have been the focus of several studies since 1990. Walters *et al.* (1990) compared

63 incontinent women with a matched control group and found that the former reported more sexual dysfunction. In a review of medical notes of 193 incontinent women aged below 60 years attending a gynaecology department, Berglund and Fugl-Meyer (1991) did not support these findings. However, they note that the study is limited to only the data recorded by the doctors and that not all doctors may have asked about sexual function nor recorded their findings. Urine loss during sexual activity was reported, however, by 34% in a questionnaire survey of 196 incontinent women (Vierhout and Gianotten, 1993) and by 56% of the 44 women in the study by Clark and Romm (1993). These studies all focused on urinary incontinence in women, and no studies were found which identified the effects of urinary incontinence on male sexual activity.

The small samples used in the ethnographic studies of women's experiences and feelings about incontinence preclude their generalisation to a wider population. However, the quality and depth of the findings add an extra dimension to the available research on incontinence, and common themes can in fact be seen to emerge from the various studies. The threat to self-esteem and a desire for normalisation emerged in most studies. Women saw it as a problem of loss of personal control and had taken steps to manage the condition and thus regain control. Self-care measures taken included regular toileting, the use of sanitary pads and restricting fluids, and a few reported doing pelvic floor exercises (Dowd, 1991; Thomas and Morse, 1991; Birgersson et al., 1993; Ashworth and Hagan, 1993; Skoner and Haylor, 1993). Ashworth and Hagan (1993) note how much effort is involved in the attempts to assure normality, and Dowd (1991) suggests that more research is needed on how to help sufferers sustain these efforts.

The effects of caring for an elderly incontinent person were measured by Flaherty et al. (1992), 22% saying that it was a burden, being associated with a lack of social support, the amount of time spent, and care required if the incontinent person was also immobile. From interviews with 184 carers of demented elderly people in the community in America, Ouslander, Zanit et al. (1990) found that 36% viewed incontinence as a problem. Incontinence was found to be a factor in the decision by carers to institutionalise demented relatives (Ouslander, Zanit et al., 1990) and was shown to be a predictor of institutionalisation (O'Donnell et al., 1992).

This review has shown that there is an emerging body of research on the effects of incontinence on individuals and that there are significant personal costs to be borne by both sufferers and carers. Wyman *et al.* (1990) concluded their review by recommending further research into the differences in psychosocial impact between the sexes and age groups and into the changes that occur in psychosocial impact following treatment. Despite the continued research into the effects of incontinence since 1990, these areas remain inadequately studied and worthy of further attention.

Causes and types of urinary incontinence

Normal bladder function

In an excellent review of the aetiology of incontinence, Cheater (1992) discusses various definitions of normal bladder function. The following definition encompasses these:

> The ability to store and void urine at will, in suitable places at convenient times and in the absence of any sensation of the need to do so and to remain continent if micturition is delayed, during exercise, standing up or sleep.

The skills involved in continence are acquired through maturation and learning during childhood and are then subconscious and automatic in most circumstances. Urinary incontinence arises when there is a breakdown in normal bladder function (Cheater, 1992). It can be caused by pathological, anatomical or physiological factors affecting the urinary tract and other areas and multiple and interacting factors can often contribute to its development (AHCPR, 1992).

Causes of urinary incontinence

The causes and types of urinary incontinence are well documented and reviewed in the literature, although, as Cheater (1992) noted, the various classifications each had their shortcomings. The standardised terminology for lower urinary tract dysfunction produced by the ICS (Andersen *et al.*, 1988) distinguished between the symptoms, signs and condition of incontinence. In the following discussion of the causes of incontinence, these standardised definitions are incorporated.

Using the model utilised by Norton (1986) and described by Cheater (1992), the causes of incontinence were classified into physiological bladder dysfunction, factors influencing bladder dysfunction and factors affecting the individual's ability to cope with the bladder.

Physiological bladder dysfunction

Detrusor instability describes the contraction of the detrusor, sponta-
neously or on provocation, during bladder filling while the patient is
attempting to inhibit micturition, demonstrated objectively (Andersen *et al.*, 1988). This term is used when the cause is idiopathic,
whereas when it is associated with a known neurological disorder, it
is called *detrusor hyperreflexia*. Symptoms most commonly associated
with detrusor instability are urgency, frequency, nocturia and urge
incontinence–an involuntary loss of urine (enuresis), which may be
nocturnal, associated with an urgent desire to void (Wall, 1990). This
is the most common cause of urinary incontinence in the elderly
(Malone-Lee, 1994).

Genuine stress incontinence is 'the involuntary loss of urine occurring
when, in the absence of a detrusor contraction, the intravesical pressure exceeds the maximum urethral pressure' (Andersen *et al.*, 1988,
p.17). This is distinguished by Andersen *et al.* (1988) from the symptom of stress incontinence when a person reports loss of urine when
coughing, exercising, etc., and the sign that denotes the observation
of involuntary loss of urine from the urethra synchronous with physical exercise. Genuine stress incontinence is the most common cause
of incontinence in women, being related to injury at childbirth
(Cardozo, 1991), and is rare in men (Cheater, 1992).

Overflow incontinence, the involuntary loss of urine because of overdistension of the bladder (Andersen *et al.*, 1988), is often caused by outflow
obstruction. Detrusor instability is also associated with outflow obstruction and an underactive bladder (Brading and Turner, 1994). Overflow
incontinence arising from outflow obstruction is most commonly
associated with prostatic enlargement, especially in men aged over 55
years, but it may also be caused by chronic constipation and urethral
stenosis or stricture. Initially, however, symptoms are likely to be hesi-
tancy, poor stream and postmicturition dribble (Cheater, 1992).

An underactive bladder arises when the detrusor muscle is underactive
and unable to sustain an adequate contraction during micturition. It
is usually caused by peripheral nerve damage and may be related to
conditions such as diabetic neuropathy, multiple sclerosis or damage
to the lower spinal cord. Overflow incontinence may eventually
occur (Cheater, 1992).

Mixed incontinence may occur when more than one of these types of physiological bladder dysfunction exists, although it is most commonly used to refer to a combination of genuine stress incontinence and detrusor instability.

Factors influencing bladder function

Transient urinary incontinence, including enuresis in children, may arise from factors that influence bladder function. These include the following:

Urinary tract infection. Cheater (1992) states that acute infection may sensitise stretch receptors in the bladder, leading to dysuria and urgency, and thus causing transient urinary incontinence. The precise role of bacteriuria in incontinence in the elderly is still unclear (Bernard, 1994). However, urinary tract infection has been strongly correlated to combined day- and night-time enuresis in 7-year-old children and to daytime wetting alone (Hansson, 1992).

Constipation and faecal impaction. This may precipitate urge or overflow incontinence by compression of the bladder and urethra (AHCPR, 1992; Cheater, 1992). Problems of faecal incontinence and constipation are associated with urinary incontinence in adults (Diokno *et al.*, 1990) and children (Maizels *et al.*, 1993).

Drug therapy. The side-effects of many drugs, several of which may be over-the-counter medications, may influence bladder function:

* *Sedative hypnotics,* especially longacting agents, may accumulate in the elderly, causing confusion and immobility and leading to secondary incontinence (AHCPR, 1992).
* *Diuretics* that produce a rapid diuresis may lead to polyuria, frequency and urge incontinence (AHCPR, 1992), particularly in patients with detrusor instability (Diokno *et al.*, 1991).
* *Anticholinergic agents* in both prescription and non-prescription medications, *anti-parkinsonian* drugs, *antidepressants* and *antispasmodics* may all cause urinary retention with overflow incontinence.
* *Alpha-adrenergic antagonists* may affect the proximal urethra by decreasing sphincter tone (e.g. prazosin) and thus cause stress incontinence in women (Dwyer and Teele, 1992).

Alpha-agonists, as found in many decongestants, could predispose older men with prostate enlargement to urinary retention by increasing sphincter tone.

- *Caffeine* is not only a diuretic but has also been shown to have an excitory effect on detrusor muscle and may exacerbate detrusor instability (Creighton and Stanton, 1990).
- *Alcohol* has a diuretic action but may also cause sedation and immobility, resulting in incontinence (AHCPR, 1992), especially nocturnal enuresis, in adults.

Endocrine disorders. These may cause or exacerbate incontinence. The polyuria associated with diabetes mellitus and diabetic insipidus could predispose to incontinence, and diabetic neuropathy can cause an underactive bladder. Postmenopausal hypo-oestrogenism affects urethral closure and lower urinary tract function (Fantl *et al.*, 1994). Studies by Norgaard and Djurhuus (1993) have shown some children suffering from nocturnal enuresis to lack the normal nocturnal increase in antidiuretic hormone levels, resulting in a higher nocturnal urine production.

The effect of ageing on bladder function. This includes hypotrophic changes in bladder smooth muscle, collagen and elastic tissue, diminished muscle tone in the bladder, urethral sphincters and pelvic muscles, and decreased bladder capacity (Houston, 1993; Bernard, 1994). Urge incontinence with reduced bladder sensation in elderly people may also be a consequence of cortical neuropathy (Griffiths *et al.*, 1994). However, Cheater (1992) notes that incontinence is not an inevitable consequence of ageing and that it often occurs only as a result of the interplay of many of these various factors.

Specific medical illness. For example, cardiovascular problems of transient ischaemic attacks and angina, and nerve and muscle disease are associated with incontinence (Diokno *et al.*, 1990). Incontinence is common in stroke patients and may be due to injury to neuromicturition pathways and/or cognitive impairment, with mobility and/or communication difficulties compounding the problem (Gelber *et al.*, 1992). Upper airway obstruction has been associated with nocturnal enuresis in children (Weider *et al.*, 1991; Maizels *et al.*, 1993).

Factors affecting the ability to cope with the bladder

Factors that influence an individual's ability to cope with a full bladder may also cause transient urinary incontinence and/or exacerbate existing incontinence, including enuresis in children.

Mobility and physical functioning have been shown to be linked to frequency of incontinence, slower mobility leading to more frequent incontinent episodes (Palmer *et al.*, 1991; Wyman *et al.*, 1993).

Environmental factors are related to mobility and include distance and access to the toilet. Cheater (1992) notes a lack of research into the extent to which environmental changes account for incontinence. Wyman *et al.* (1993) studied frequency of incontinence in relation to distance to the nearest toilet in elderly people residing in the community and found that the nearer the toilet, the more frequent the episodes of incontinence. This is obviously contrary to what might have been expected and deserves further study. Other environmental factors, such as chair height, clothing and mobility aids, will contribute to the maintenance of continence (Turner-Stokes and Frank, 1992; Roe and Williams, 1994). Bedtime routines and access to the toilet at night may influence nocturnal enuresis in children (Clark *et al.*, 1994).

Mental state has been linked to incontinence through studies that have shown dementia to be positively correlated with incontinence (McGrother *et al.*, 1990; Palmer *et al.*, 1991; Ouslander *et al.*, 1993). Depression and anxiety have been associated with incontinence (Macaulay *et al.*, 1991), although whether this is a cause or effect is unclear.

Developmental factors for example, people with learning difficulties may have problems with toileting. Nocturnal enuresis is more common in children with learning difficulties (Smith and Smith, 1987).

Psychological factors such as bereavement and institutionalisation may be linked to incontinence (Cheater, 1992). Children living in institutions show a greater tendency to suffer from enuresis (Butler, 1994). Other factors such as anxiety, depression and psychoneuroticism have been implicated in the aetiology of incontinence (Macaulay *et al.*, 1991), but their precise role is unclear and some studies have found no relationship (Moore and Sutherst, 1990; Norton *et al.*, 1990; Lagro-Janssen, Debruyne and van Weel, 1992).

Carers' attitudes and actions may have an influence on incontinence, especially if negative attitudes are displayed (Cheater, 1992). Parental and family attitudes are important factors in the treatment of children with enuresis (Maizels *et al.*, 1993; Butler, 1994).

Risk factors related to urinary incontinence

In addition to the factors described that may cause incontinence, studies have identified risk factors that may indicate a person's susceptibility to developing incontinence. There is obvious overlap with those factors already described, which, by their nature as causative factors, are also risk factors.

Other risk factors identified from the literature for adults include:

* smoking;
* pregnancy;
* parity;
* body mass index;
* race;
* previous surgery;
* family history of childhood bedwetting;
* childhood bedwetting;
* exercise.

Table 4.2 summarises the studies published since 1990 that demonstrated positive links between the various risk factors and urinary incontinence in adults. However, the evidence for these links is in most cases correlational and in some cases not statistically proven. Other studies (e.g. Burgio *et al.*, 1991) have found no relationship between smoking, parity, previous surgery and incontinence. There is a need for further research using standardised definitions of incontinence and methodologies to examine the risk factors in more detail, since accurate identification may help to prevent the occurrence of incontinence as well as aid its treatment.

In children, a family history of bedwetting and the occurrence of stressful events in early life were definite risk factors for nocturnal enuresis (Devlin, 1991; Clark *et al.*, 1994). Family attitudes and parental intolerance were risk factors involved in both day- and night-time wetting in children. Children of lower socio-economic groups and from large families living in overcrowded conditions were also more at risk of enuresis (Butler, 1994).

Table 4.2: Summary of studies since 1990 demonstrating positive links between risk factors and urinary incontinence

Risk factor and study	Method	Results and conclusions
Smoking		
Bump and McClish (1992)	Case control study, 322 incontinent women compared with 284 continent women	Risk of GSI was strongly correlated with the intensity of smoking and lifetime exposure to smoking. Results statistically significant
Bump and McClish (1994)	Case control study of 189 women with GSI: 118 smokers and 71 non-smokers had urodynamic evaluation	Smokers with GSI were younger than non-smokers ($p = 0.002$). Smokers generate greater bladder pressure increases with coughing ($p = 0.05$). More violent coughing by smokers probably promotes earlier development of GSI
Race		
Burgio *et al.* (1991)	Prevalence study of 486 women aged 42–50 in Pittsburgh, USA by interview and physical examination	White women more likely to report regular incontinence than black. Statistically significant
Bump (1993)	Prospective evaluation of 200 women 54 of whom were black, referred for evaluation of urinary incontinence or severe prolapse	Black women with urinary incontinence have a different distribution of symptoms, conditions causing their incontinence and risk profiles than white women. Results statistically significant. More research needed
Exercise		
Nygaard *et al.* (1994)	Questionnaire survey of 144 women: nulliparous, college athletes	Incontinence during sport reported by 28%. UI is common in young, fit, nulliparous women. There may be a threshold, which when exceeded can result in urine loss even in absence of known risk factors. No statistical testing

(contd)

Table 4.2: (contd)

Risk factor and study	Method	Results and conclusions
Body mass index Burgio et al. (1991)	Prevalence study of 486 women aged 42–50 in Pittsburgh, USA, by interview and physical examination	Statistically significant relationship between body mass index and all types of UI. Weight gain may increase susceptibility to UI and weight loss may reduce UI
Bump et al. (1992)	Subjective and objective evaluation of lower urinary tract function measured before and 1 year after surgically induced weight loss in 13 morbidly obese women	Statistically significant improvements ($p = 0.004$) of lower urinary tract function after weight loss. Objective and subjective resolution of urge and stress incontinence. Weight reduction is desirable for severely obese women and may reduce need for further incontinence therapy. Small sample
Simeonova and Bengtsson (1990)	Prevalence questionnaire survey of women aged 18 and over visiting Swedish health centre ($N = 451$)	Women with body mass index > 25kg/m² reported significantly more UI than those whose body mass was below this level. Data on 115 women were missing
Pregnancy Diokno et al. (1990)	Probability sample of residents aged 60 and over of Washentaw County, Michigan, USA, interviewed in their homes ($N = 1956$; response rate 65%)	Incontinence during or immediately after pregnancy was found to correlate highly with UI in later life, especially stress incontinence. Pregnancy itself did not correlate with UI
Viktrup et al. (1992)	Prospective study of 305 primiparae, interviewed about stress UI before, during and after pregnancy	4% had stress UI before pregnancy, 32% during, 21% developed it after delivery, 3% still had stress UI 1 year after delivery, all with onset during or after pregnancy. Pregnancy carries a small (1% or less) risk of initiating persistent stress UI. Statistical significance unclear

Study	Description	Findings
Foldspang et al. (1992)	Cross-sectional prevalence study of UI in 1987 of 2613 women aged 30–59 in Aarhus, Denmark, using postal questionnaire. Also includes a review and bivariate reanalysis of other published studies	Re-analysis of earlier studies concludes that there are mutually conflicting findings with regard to the influence of parity on UI. Strong statistically significant relationship found between parity and the development and persistence of UI, especially stress UI. Prevalence of UI increased with parity and was associated with age at last childbirth
Molander (1993)	Prevalence study of stratified sample of women aged 46–85 in Gothenburg, Sweden ($N = 7459$)	Prevalence of UI strongly correlated to parity, increase being most apparent after birth of first child
Harrison and Memel (1994)	Postal questionnaire prevalence survey of random sample of women aged 20 years and over in one general practice in Bristol, UK ($N = 384$)	Positive correlation between childbirth and incontinence, but no link between UI and mode of delivery, baby's weight or perineal suturing
Childhood bedwetting Moore et al. (1991)	Retrospective review of urodynamic case records of 1000 men and women and analysis of links with childhood bedwetting in 198 with idiopathic detrusor instability	History of childhood nocturnal enuresis was significantly more common in men than women. Of all patients with a bedwetting history, 76% of men and 61% of women were found to have unstable bladders
Foldspang and Mommsen (1994)	Cross-sectional prevalence study of UI in 1987 in 2613 women aged 30–59 in Aarhus, Denmark, using postal questionnaire	Childhood bedwetting was associated with prevalent urge incontinence ($p<0.01$) and incontinence during sleep ($p<0.0001$). Some individuals may suffer a long-lasting disturbance of balance between micturition and sleep processes

(contd)

Table 4.2: (contd)

Risk factor and study	Method	Results and conclusions
Previous surgery Diokno *et al.* (1990)	Probability sample of residents aged 60 and over of Washentaw County, Michigan, USA interviewed in homes ($N = 1956$; response rate 65%)	Incontinent respondents reported significantly more surgery, including genital and rectal but excluding incontinence-related surgery, than continent respondents
Mommsen *et al.* (1993)	Cross-sectional prevalence study of UI in 1987 in 2613 women aged 30–59 in Aarhus, Denmark, using postal questionnaire	Stress urinary incontinence was associated with previous exposure to surgery, especially gynaecological surgery. Statistically significant

GSI = genuine stress incontinence;   UI = urinary incontinence.

Additionally, various factors may predict response to treatment for nocturnal enuresis in children, these including family and social factors as well as behavioural factors in the child (Butler, 1991).

Assessment of urinary incontinence and enuresis

The literature on assessment has been reviewed with particular reference to the role of the PHCT. The review has focused on the assessment to be undertaken by the PHCT and the circumstances in which referral for further tests such as urodynamic testing should take place. Details of the various urodynamic tests are not therefore reviewed.

Within the literature review, it was apparent that there was agreement that all patients reporting urinary incontinence including children should be assessed (Brocklehurst, 1990a; Resnick, 1990a, b; AHCPR, 1992; Duffin, 1992; Walters and Realini, 1992; Maizels *et al.*, 1993; Rushton, 1993). Studies have shown that fewer than 50% of patients report urinary incontinence symptoms to their doctors (Devlin, 1991; O'Brien *et al.*, 1991; Goldstein *et al.*, 1992; Hunskaar, 1992; Brocklehurst, 1993; Sandvik *et al.*, 1993, Harrison and Memel, 1994; Rappuport, 1994). It was therefore also recommended that, in order to identify such patients, routine open questions relating to 'bladder problems' or 'problems with passing water' were directed to patients when presenting to the PHCT (AHCPR, 1992; Duffin, 1992), for example during screening for the over 75-year-olds, at Well Man/Woman clinics, during cervical cytology screening and in school medicals.

Assessment

There was considerable consensus on what should comprise the assessment, although this did not appear to be based on empirical evidence. The assessment is described in detail elsewhere (Brocklehurst, 1990a; Resnick, 1990a, b; Duffin, 1992; Walters and Realini, 1992; Houston, 1993; Morgan, 1993; Rushton, 1993; Bernard, 1994; Clark *et al.*, 1994; Roe and Williams, 1994; Blackwell, 1995), and therefore only a summary of the assessment is presented here. This assessment may be undertaken over a period of time, and a sensitive and supportive approach is necessary (Duffin, 1992). A supportive relationship between health care professional and parent and child has been shown to be an important factor in the successful treatment of enuresis (Clark *et al.*, 1994).

History

A detailed history should be taken of the symptoms of incontinence or wetting, the characteristics, duration, frequency, severity, precipitants, associated symptoms and effects on the quality of life of the individual/carer, including effects on sexual activity if appropriate. Details of aids used and self-care measures taken should be recorded. A family history concerning childhood bedwetting should be taken. Medical, surgical, neurological, genitourinary and obstetric histories and a review of medications, including non-prescription drugs, are required in order to identify any related illnesses or causes. Bowel function should also be reviewed, including control of flatus, as faecal impaction may lead to incontinence and incontinence of flatus can indicate weak pelvic floor musculature, particularly in women. The type and amount of fluid intake should be assessed; for example, caffeine, alcohol or a high fluid intake at bedtime may all exacerbate incontinence. A review of functional abilities and developmental and environmental factors may also identify causes of incontinence.

For children, the history should also include the attitudes of the parents and the child to the wetting and the family reaction. Funtional payoffs when wetting occurs, e.g. sleeping in the parents' bed and cuddles from parents, should be considered.

Physical examination

Height, weight and body mass index are required. Abdominal examination should be undertaken in adults and children. Physical examination should include examination of the perineum, genital examination in men, pelvic examination in women, rectal examination and general examination for neurological abnormalities or other precipitating conditions. Assessment of general mobility and physical functioning is important in the elderly.

Urinalysis

Urine should be tested using dipsticks for routine urinalysis, and midstream urine should be taken for culture and sensitivity and red blood cells in both adults and children.

Assessment charts

Frequency/volume charts should be completed by the patient for up to 1 week in order to identify usual micturition patterns and may also incorporate fluid intake.

Estimation of post-voiding residual urine

This can be estimated by abdominal palpation and percussion or measured specifically by catheterisation (Duffin, 1992) or pelvic ultrasound (Revord *et al.*, 1993).

Provocative stress test

This is recommended if stress incontinence is suspected.

Other tests that may be initiated by the PHCT include abdominal X-ray, urine cytology and blood tests for metabolic disturbances (Duffin, 1992).

Evaluation by urodynamic studies

Whilst there is consensus on the composition of an initial assessment, there is considerable debate in the literature concerning the need for further evaluation of urinary incontinence through urodynamic testing in order for the clinician to make a diagnosis.

The ICS definition (Andersen *et al.*, 1988) of urinary incontinence refers to its 'objective demonstration' and suggests that it cannot be diagnosed without urodynamic evaluation. In efforts to determine whether or not such testing is required to make a diagnosis, several studies have attempted to measure the correlation between patients' histories of their incontinence and their urodynamic diagnosis. In most cases, the conclusions were that diagnosis cannot be made on the evidence of patients' symptoms alone and that urodynamic testing was essential (Bergman and Bader, 1990; LeCoutour *et al.*, 1990; Versi *et al.*, 1991; Summitt *et al.*, 1992).

Indeed, Jensen *et al.* (1994), in a meta-analysis of 19 out of 29 articles published between 1975 and 1992 comparing patient history with urodynamic testing, concluded that patient history alone is not an accurate tool in the diagnosis of genuine stress incontinence or detrusor overactivity. However, Resnick (1990b) and Lagro-Janssen, Debruyne and van Weel (1991) pointed out that most of these studies were undertaken on patients referred for urodynamic testing and for hospital treatment. They argue that these samples probably include more complex cases than those seen in routine general practice. The studies also all referred to adults rather than children. The study by Bergman and Bader (1990) of 122 women did, however, include a control group of 32 continent females with no urinary incontinence. This study concluded that history alone can be misleading in diagnosing urinary incontinence.

Despite this evidence concerning the potential weaknesses of diagnosing urinary incontinence in the absence of urodynamic testing, several authors argue that GPs are able to make an initial diagnosis and commence therapy in the majority of cases (Brocklehurst, 1990a; Resnick, 1990a, b; Lagro-Janssen, Debruyne and van Weel, 1991; Walters and Realini, 1992; Houston, 1993; Bernard, 1994). The arguments given in favour of this approach included the high prevalence of urinary incontinence and the lack of sufficient available urodynamic facilities, the costs and time required for testing and the fact that tests are uncomfortable, especially for elderly people. However, with the exception of Lagro-Janssen, Debruyne and van Weel (1990), who were studying women aged 20–65 years, all these authors were referring to the care of the elderly person with urinary incontinence. Resnick (1990b) points out, however, that many earlier studies were concerned with diagnostic accuracy in younger females.

There is, therefore, no consensus on the requirement for all patients to undergo urodynamic testing in order for a diagnosis to be made. In some instances, criteria have been given that determine which individuals should be referred for further testing, including:

1. If the diagnosis is unclear, especially where there is a lack of correlation between symptomatology and clinical findings (Resnick, 1990; AHCPR, 1992; Walters and Realini, 1992).
2. When the risk of a trial therapy is unacceptable (Resnick, 1990a).
3. When initial therapy has failed (Resnick, 1990a; AHCPR, 1992; Walters and Realini, 1992).
4. The presence of other co-morbid conditions, e.g. recurrent urinary tract infections, neurological conditions or a prostate nodule.
5. Prior to referral for surgery (Bernard, 1994).
6. In the presence of marked pelvic prolapse (AHCPR, 1992; Bernard, 1994).
7. In cases of severe stress incontinence (Bernard, 1994).
8. With an abnormal post-voiding residual urine volume (AHCPR, 1992; Bernard, 1994).
9. When there is microhaematuria without infection (AHCPR, 1992; Walters and Realini, 1992; Bernard, 1994; Clark et al., 1994).

In addition, children with enuresis should be referred in the following instances (Clark et al., 1994; RCP, 1995):

• abnormal physical examination;

- daytime wetting and voiding symptoms;
- abnormalities on urinalysis and positive signs of infection on a midstream specimen of urine;
- major bowel disturbance and severe encopresis;
- adverse parameters predicting poor response and compliance;
- nocturnal enuresis in the schoolage child not responding to an alarm/drugs.

On the basis of the literature review, it is not possible to determine whether or not urodynamic studies are required on all patients. The use of criteria such as those presented here would, however, facilitate the determination of the need for such testing and would enable the GP or other member of the PHCT to undertake an initial assessment and initiate therapy in the majority of cases of urinary incontinence. There is obviously a need for further discussion and research in order to clarify these issues. Further research evidence is also required to substantiate the consensus view of the composition of an assessment.

Promotion/restoration of continence

The aim of the treatment and care of patients suffering from urinary incontinence is for the person to regain continence. Treatments that aim to promote or restore continence include behavioural therapy, surgery and drug therapy (AHCPR, 1992).

Behavioural therapy

Behavioural techniques include bladder and pelvic muscle re-education programmes as well as biofeedback techniques and conditioning methods. These are considered separately, although many studies have utilised a combination of these, often in conjunction with drug therapy.

Bladder re-education

Bladder re-education programmes aim to restore continence either by re-educating the bladder to a normal or improved pattern of continence or by avoiding incontinence episodes through prompted voiding at planned times. Patients with urgency, urge incontinence and detrusor instability are most likely to benefit from these programmes (Roe and Williams, 1994), although patients suffering from stress incontinence have also been shown to benefit (AHCPR, 1992). Meadows (1990), Maizels *et al.* (1993) and Clark *et al.* (1994) have described various bladder re-education techniques that have been used successfully with children suffering from daytime wetting.

Four types of programme are generally described in the literature, based on work by Hadley (1986). These are distinguished by the type of voiding schedule employed, i.e. bladder training, habit training, timed voiding or prompted voiding (Kennedy, 1992). Each is now briefly described, along with details of recent research.

Bladder training. The time interval between voiding is progressively increased. Intervals are mandatory or self-adjusted. Patients need to be motivated and able both physically and mentally to toilet themselves (Hadley, 1986). Meadows (1990) and Maizels *et al.* (1993) reported that studies using this technique with children have had fair success in treating enuresis.

Fantl *et al.* (1990) demonstrated improvements in the number of incontinence episodes, the quantity of urine loss and associated symptoms in a randomised controlled trial of bladder training with 123 non-institutionalised women aged 55 years or over. Objective and subjective measures were used and 12% of women were cured, and a total of 75% improving by 50% or more. McDowell *et al.* (1992) used bladder training in conjunction with pelvic floor exercises with 70 non-demented community-dwelling elderly people. The mean reduction in the frequency of accidents reported was 82%. Burgio (1990) reported on a study whereby a nurse practitioner ran a bladder training programme for elderly persons in a geriatric outpatient department and achieved an 80% reduction in accidents. Burgio concluded that bladder training offers a low-risk treatment with an absence of documented side-effects that is a useful treatment in situations when surgery or drug therapy is contraindicated or unwanted, especially in the elderly. A 2-year study involving 115 patients with symptoms of frequency, urgency and urge incontinence was undertaken by Hyland (1991). Patients were seen every 2–3 weeks by the continence adviser and every 2–3 months in a joint clinic with a urologist. Eighty-nine per cent of patients reported cures; however, there were no control groups and treatments were mixed.

Improvements in the continence status of patients treated by GPs or nurses in a general practice, using bladder training, were found by O'Brien *et al.* (1991), Lagro-Janssen, Debruyne, Smits *et al.* (1992) and Harrison and Memel (1994). Lagro-Janssen, Debruyne, Smits *et al.* (1992)

successfully treated 110 females aged 65 years or less with simple incontinence using pelvic floor exercises and bladder training. Seventy-four per cent felt that their condition had improved, and this improvement was reflected in a severity index. In the randomised controlled study by O'Brien *et al.* (1991), a non-specialist nurse treated 292 women and 22 men using bladder training and pelvic floor exercises. Sixty-eight per cent of the women reported cure or improvement, and 17 out of the 22 men were cured. No objective measures were, however, used to assess improvements.

McClish *et al.* (1991) implemented a bladder training protocol with 108 women but found very few urodynamic changes 6 weeks later. Nonetheless, 50% of subjects reported a reduction in the number of incontinent episodes. No control group was used. McClish *et al.* (1991) concluded that bladder training may reflect behavioural changes rather than physiological changes, although Kennedy (1992) said that earlier studies that used objective measures had demonstrated urodynamic improvement.

The efficacy of bladder training in improving subjective measures of incontinence is demonstrated by the subjects in these studies. The actual mechanism involved in the improvement, be it behavioural or physiological, needs further study. The role of the nurse and GP in bladder training programmes has been shown to be effective, although further studies using controls, standardised terminology, objective measures and longer periods of follow-up would enhance the evidence.

Habit training. The time between voiding is altered to suit the individual's voiding pattern, either increased or decreased. This method is suitable for patients who may have mental or physical disabilities and requires motivated staff (Kennedy, 1992). The AHCPR (1992) clinical guideline does not distinguish between habit training and timed voiding. No recent research studies relating to the approach of habit training as described here were found.

Timed voiding. This involves scheduled voiding to a rigid regime. It is often used for debilitated elderly people, usually with a 2-hourly interval (Kennedy, 1992). It is also used for patients with a neurogenic bladder, often in conjunction with triggers such as running water or tapping the thigh, and was successfully used to treat 55 spinal cord injury patients in a study by Menon and Tan (1992).

Prompted voiding. This method is used most often with institutionalised patients. It utilises a fixed prompting schedule but a varying voiding schedule, as follows. Patients are asked whether they wish to void at regular intervals but are only taken to the toilet if they want to go. Positive reinforcement is used to encourage patients. Studies by Schnelle (1990), Colling *et al.* (1992) and Burgio *et al.* (1994) all demonstrated reductions in incontinent episodes when prompted voiding was introduced in institutional settings with the elderly. Colling *et al.* (1992) reported that some patients felt more in control and pleased with the approach. Burgio *et al.* (1994) were able to demonstrate continued improvements once patients returned from the continence unit to their usual units.

There is, therefore, evidence that bladder re-education is an effective means of treatment for the promotion of continence. However, Cheater (1991b) found a lack of consensus in the use of terminology related to bladder re-education programmes even amongst continence advisers. She also pointed out the use of poorly defined methods with few controls in research studies related to these programmes, as did Kennedy (1992) in her review of studies up until 1990. Kennedy concluded that research shows that bladder re-education can cure or improve continence for those subjects participating in trials, but the programmes require motivated individuals and may take up to 3 months to show effect. However, as Kennedy concluded in 1992, there is still a need for further research to understand how bladder re-education works and for larger randomly controlled trials of bladder re-education programmes, with and without other forms of treatment, as well as for longer follow-up periods.

Behavioural techniques for nocturnal enuresis

A critical review of the literature on diagnosis and treatment for children who cannot control urination by Maizels *et al.* (1993) described several studies demonstrating success using enuresis alarms with children and concluded that this is the most successful treatment for nocturnal enuresis. Around 60–80% of children using an alarm have been shown to attain dryness within 2–4 months of commencing treatment (Gustafson, 1993; Butler, 1994; Clark *et al.*, 1994). However, success depended on patient selection, education, enthusiasm and the choice of an appropriate alarm. Alarms may be body-worn or of the pad and buzzer type (Clark *et al.*, 1994), and patients should be offered a choice (Morgan, 1993). Minimum standards for the use of enuretic alarms have been produced by ERIC (Morgan, 1993).

Other conditioning methods, e.g. dry bed training and overlearning therapy, have been shown to increase the success with alarm therapy. Van Londen *et al.* (1993) found that, in a 2½-year follow-up of 113 children aged 6–12 years suffering from nocturnal enuresis, arousal therapy used in conjunction with alarm therapy was the most successful treatment. Reinforcements such as star charts may also be used to reward achievement of compliance with the training task rather than continence itself.

Enuresis alarms are also useful in adults. McCormick *et al.* (1992) used an electronic bell pad to aid prompted voiding in elderly people, achieving a 22% improvement in dryness, although no control was used and sample size was small.

Behaviour therapy techniques

These techniques, based on operant conditioning and the use of rewards, have been shown to be effective in improving toileting behaviour and continence in individuals with learning difficulties (Smith and Smith, 1987; Roe, 1992b).

Pelvic floor muscle re-education

The muscles of the pelvic floor provide elasticity and strength in supporting the abdominal and pelvic organs. Weakness of these muscles and/or damage to their nerve supply can result in prolapse of the pelvic organs and weakness of the urinary sphincter, and can cause urinary and faecal incontinence. Allen *et al.* (1990) showed that obstetric trauma may damage the pudendal nerves. Childbirth, reduced activity, increasing age, obesity and trauma can all reduce the strength and elasticity of the muscles. However, this can be regained and restored in many cases through pelvic muscle exercises and electrical stimulation (Laycock, 1992).

Pelvic floor muscle re-education is generally used for women with stress incontinence as an initial therapy, and, compared with surgery, it is significantly less costly, both financially and physiologically (Brubaker and Kotarinos, 1993). It is also used for women who have had multiple surgical repairs and for men following prostatectomy (Roe and Williams, 1994). Pelvic muscle exercises have been used successfully for urge incontinence (Flynn *et al.*, 1994) and even for children experiencing day- and night-time wetting (Schneider *et al.*, 1994). In both of these cases, however, the research evidence is small.

Laycock (1992) provided an excellent review of pelvic muscle re-education and recommended that all patients required a digital assessment to check whether they are contracting the correct muscles and also to evaluate the effects of exercise. This is especially important since Bump *et al.* (1991) found that women who are given verbal instructions alone may adopt a technique for contraction of the pelvic muscles that actually promotes the defect responsible for their incontinence. A grading system is recommended and is described in detail by Laycock (1992). The use of the grading system enables individualised programmes of exercise to be determined for each patient.

The effectiveness of pelvic muscle re-education is discussed by Williams *et al.* (1995). Table 4.3 is reproduced from this study, with the authors' permission, since it provides a comprehensive account of recent research studies. Williams *et al.* (1995) concluded that studies varied in their design, the exercise programmes implemented, the person undertaking the training programme and the measures used to test effectiveness.

Comparisons of these results were therefore difficult, although cure or improvement ranged from 47% to 77%. Williams *et al.* (1995) noted that only three studies in Table 4.3 looked at the long-term effects of pelvic muscle re-education. Dougherty *et al.* (1993) used two follow-up surveys for 65 women aged 35–75 who had participated in a trial programme of pelvic muscle re-education. They contacted the subjects from 8 to 26 months after completion of the programme. On each survey, approximately 10% of women indicated that their incontinence had increased since the study had ended. Dougherty *et al.* (1993) argue that, as 90% had not deteriorated, this supports the value of pelvic muscle re-education without additional input from a therapist. However, there is the need, as identified by Bump *et al.* (1991), continually to ensure that women are performing the exercise correctly. Such support could be provided by nurses or physiotherapists, although a study by Mantle and Versi (1991) involving physiotherapists from 192 district health authorities found that treatments varied considerably. They recommended research to determine the most cost-effective management of stress incontinence since the majority of women whom the physiotherapists were treating were also the best candidates for surgery.

In conclusion, there is consensus that pelvic muscle re-education is widely used and that it has a place in the promotion of continence, is of low risk if taught adequately and has been shown to improve stress incontinence, at least in the short term. More research is needed, however, on the long-term effects, the optimum treatment pattern and the motivational support required by patients.

Table 4.3: Studies of pelvic floor muscle exercises

Authors	Design	Sample	Method	Measures	Findings
Sleep and Grant (1987)	Two-group RCT	1800 inpatients Mean age = 26	Individual instruction in PME, urinary diary. Control = traditional PME	Objective Subjective	No difference between traditional and individualised PME
Peattie et al. (1988)	Single group	N = 39 Mean age = 38	Taught use of vaginal cones to exercise PM 15 min twice per day	Objective Subjective	70% cure or improvement
Cammu et al. (1991)	Prospective cohort study	N = 52 Mean age = 53	PME by physio twice per week for 10 weeks	Objective Subjective	25% cure, high report of improvement, less demand for surgery
Wells et al. (1991)	Two group	N = 157 Mean age = 66	Group 1 verbal inst 90–160 PME per day Group 2 drug therapy	Objective Subjective	Cure or improvement 77% Group 1 84% Group 2
Mouritsen et al. (1991)	Single group	N = 100 Mean age = 53	Weekly physio sessions of 45 min for 3 month PME programme	Objective Subjective	47% cure or improvement
Lagro-Janssen, Debruyne, Smits et al. (1991)	RCT	N = 66 Mean age = 44	PME instructions by one GP 10 sessions of 10 contractions per day	Objective Subjective	60% cure or improvement

(contd)

Table 4.3: (contd)

Authors	Design	Sample	Method	Measures	Findings
Elia and Bergman (1993)	Single group	$N = 53$ Mean age = 59	Training by physio for 1.5 hr × 2 per week for 6 weeks + PME at home for 15 min × 4 per day	Objective Subjective	56% cure or improvement
Hahn et al. (1993)	Two groups	$N = 205$ Mean age = 52	PFE programme by physio: various times	Objective Subjective	64% cure or improvement 2–7 years later 55% still cured or improved

Reproduced with kind permission of Williams et al., 1995.
PME = pelvic muscle exercise; PM = pelvic muscle; RCT = randomised controlled trial; PFE = pelvic floor exercise.

Vaginal cones

The use of vaginal cones, which are weighted cones, was introduced by Plevnik in 1985 and may serve as an adjunct to pelvic muscle re-education in women. The cone is inserted intravaginally, and the women attempts to retain it by contracting the pelvic muscles for up to 15 minutes. In addition to increasing the strength of the pelvic muscle, this also provides proprioceptive feedback for the woman on the desired muscle contraction (Laycock, 1992; AHCPR, 1992). Brubaker and Kotarinos (1993) recommended the use of cones for women who can stop the flow of urine midstream and who can contract the correct muscles.

However, there have been few studies measuring the efficacy of the cones as a treatment for incontinence. Williams *et al.* (1995) reviewed the studies to date and found that an improvement in continence, both objective and subjective, was demonstrated in over 60% of cases. However, they caution that the number of studies and the number of subjects involved were very small.

There is a definite need for further research in this area using randomly controlled trials with larger samples. The applicability of this as a treatment to other populations, e.g. postmenopausal women with vaginal atrophy, also needs evaluation.

Electrical stimulation

The use of electrical stimulation in the treatment of incontinence is described in detail by Laycock (1992). The use of this mode of treatment has increased in recent years for both urge and stress incontinence, partly because of the introduction of portable electrical simulators that can be taken home by the patients (Roe and Williams, 1994).

The technique has been used in both neurologically and non-neurologically impaired individuals to manage both bladder and urethral dysfunction (AHCPR, 1992). Studies have shown an improvement in incontinence, but these have varied with regard to the actual conditions concerning the electrical stimulation, e.g. frequency, duration and amplitude of voltage, continuous, intermittent or phasic, so generalisations and comparisons are difficult (Fossberg *et al.*, 1990; Esa *et al.*, 1991; Hahn *et al.*, 1991; Meyer *et al.*, 1992; Zöllner-Nielsen and Samuelson, 1992; Caputo *et al.*, 1993; Schiotz, 1994).

Caputo *et al.* (1993) and Moore (1994) conclude that further research is needed using standard parameters of stimulation as are randomised controlled trials comparing the efficacy of electrical stimulation either alone or in combination with other treatments. The AHCPR (1992) guideline panel concluded that research should be undertaken before this technique becomes an established treatment for urinary incontinence, and this situation does not appear to have changed.

Biofeedback

Biofeedback has been used in the management of urinary incontinence for patients with detrusor instability (O'Donnell and Doyle, 1991) and for pelvic floor rehabilitation (Laycock and Jerwood, 1994). It has also been used with children (Maizels *et al.*, 1993). The technique relies on electronic or mechanical instruments to provide feedback to the individual about their physiological activity. It should be used in conjunction with other behavioural techniques and requires a knowledgeable and skilled health care provider (AHCPR, 1992).

Knight and Laycock (1994) described the use of biofeedback as an adjunct to pelvic floor exercises and argued that sophisticated equipment facilitates the teaching of pelvic muscle exercises. However, from their review of the literature, they could find few controlled trials which could demonstrate that exercise combined with biofeedback was more effective than exercise alone. However, a randomised controlled trial by Burns *et al.* (1993) compared biofeedback with pelvic muscle exercise alone and a control in 135 women. They found significant improvements in both treatment groups but no significant difference in the improvements between treatments. Laycock and Jerwood's (1994) conclusion that, although this form of therapy is widely available in the USA and France, further controlled studies are needed in this country to justify the cost of the equipment required, would seem to be upheld.

Surgery

Since this review is considering the promotion of continence by the PHCT literature relating to specific surgical techniques has not been included. The AHCPR guideline makes recommendations about surgical treatments for urinary incontinence (AHCPR, 1992). Recent reviews of surgical techniques for incontinence are provided by Dorsey and Cundiff (1994) and Jarvis (1994). The review of research related to surgery for stress incontinence by Jarvis (1994) demonstrated the poor comparative nature of such studies and the dearth of randomised controlled trials of techniques. He concluded that there is no single operation that should be offered to all women as a first choice for stress incontinence. The need for methodological improvements in trials of surgical techniques was highlighted.

Drug therapy

Drug therapy available for the treatment of urinary incontinence is usually categorised according to the condition to be treated; hence drugs will be considered in relation to the treatment of detrusor instability and stress incontinence. A brief mention will be made of drug therapy for nocturnal enuresis in children.

However, in all cases, there were few published randomly controlled trials on which to make judgements regarding the true efficacy of the drugs, and published trials were inadequate in many aspects (AHCPR, 1992). The review of research studies included in the AHCPR (1992) guideline on urinary incontinence in adults was the most recent evidence of the research basis for drug therapy for incontinence found in this search and is therefore referred to here with updated material where relevant. The papers by Andersson (1988) and Wein (1990) provided a thorough review of the pharmacological aspects of this therapy. For details of the availability of the various drugs in the United Kingdom, recommended dosages and details of side-effects and contraindications, readers are directed to recent editions of the *British National Formulary*, since it is not the intention of this review to cover such details.

Drugs used for the treatment of detrusor instability

The drugs used to treat detrusor instability fall into four categories:

Anticholinergic agents. These drugs block the contraction of normal bladder muscle and to some extent the unstable bladder.

Propantheline is the anticholinergic most used; it is inexpensive and has been extensively used in the USA for incontinence (AHCPR, 1992). However, the AHCPR panel found only five adequately controlled trials involving propantheline, and no other more recent studies were found in this review. Despite the lack of research evidence, the use of propantheline was recommended for less impaired patients who can tolerate full doses (AHCPR, 1992).

Antispasmodics. Oxybutynin has both smooth muscle relaxant and anticholinergic effects. Six randomised controlled trials involving adults were identified by the AHCPR panel, of which five demonstrated oral oxybutynin's superiority to placebo in reducing incontinence frequency, all in middle-aged outpatients. Oxybutynin was found to be ineffective in the one randomised controlled trial involving chronically disabled elderly described by the AHCPR panel (AHCPR, 1992). However, details of a randomised double blind trial of oxybutynin with bladder training and bladder training and a placebo in 60 frail, elderly men, of age 82 years were given by Malone-Lee (1994). The study found that oxybutynin was superior to the placebo, causing a significantly greater reduction in total frequency but no significant difference in nocturia.

No other recent trials were identified, but three studies were found that reported the use of the intravesical instillation of oxybutynin in conjunction with self-intermittent catheterisation in adults (Prasad and Vaidyanathan, 1993; Weese *et al.*, 1993; Mizunaga *et al.*, 1994) and one in children (Greenfield and Fera, 1991). The study by Weese *et al.* (1993) involved 42 patients who were incontinent secondary to uninhibited detrusor contractions and who had failed oral anticholinergic therapy. Fifty-five per cent of the 33 patients who completed the trial experienced a significant improvement of their incontinence. The other studies involved patients with neurogenic bladders.

Whilst the AHCPR (1992) guideline recommended the use of oral oxybutynin for adults, intravesical administration is not mentioned. Further evidence of the efficacy of this route is necessary. Evidence of the efficacy of oxybutynin in children is also required since Maizels *et al.* (1993) note a lack of consensus on its benefits and point out that the only double blind controlled study found no difference between oxybutynin and placebo.

Dicyclomine hydrochloride was identified by the AHCPR panel as another anticholinergic with smooth muscle relaxant properties. Although only two randomised controlled trials were reported, one was only a pilot study and the other lacked data on statistical significance and side-effects, the panel recommended the use of this drug as an alternative to other acceptable anticholinergic agents.

Calcium channel blocking agents. The blockage of extracellular calcium by calcium agonists can reduce contraction of the bladder muscle. Such drugs include nifedipine, diltiazem, verapamil and flunarizine. From the lack of sufficient adequate research data on the use of these drugs, the AHCPR (1992) panel concluded that they should not be recommended for general use for detrusor instability. No additional research data have been found to alter this recommendation.

The drug terodiline, which is identified by the AHCPR panel as an anticholinergic and calcium channel blocking drug, has been withdrawn from use owing to the serious side-effect of ventricular arrythmia.

Tricyclic agents. The AHCPR guideline notes that drugs such as imipramine, desipramine and nortriptyline were widely used but that there were only three randomised controlled trials. Side-effects were also noted in two of the studies (AHCPR, 1992).

Only one double blind cross-over study was found, which involved a very small sample of only 13 patients with advanced multiple sclerosis. Side-effects were few and frequency diminished significantly (Kinn and Larsson, 1990).

The conclusion of the AHCPR guideline panel was to recommend the use of imipramine and doxepin in adults. Details of the randomised controlled trials in children were not available, but Maizels *et al.* (1993) reported that imipramine has been used successfully for children with nocturnal enuresis. Clark *et al.* (1994) did not, however, recommend the use of this drug in children, and Maizels *et al.* (1993) drew attention to the potential toxicity of the drug in children.

Other drugs. The use of flavoxate a tertiary amine, was not recommended as four randomised controlled trials had not demonstrated a significant benefit (AHCPR, 1992). Various other drugs were identified as having been used for detrusor instability, but the guideline did not recommend their use owing to limited studies and lack of clinical evidence.

Summary. The evidence presented by the AHCPR panel in relation to the research basis of drug therapy for detrusor instability does not appear to have changed very much since 1992. Their conclusions therefore remain valid. These included the following points (AHCPR, 1992):

- Regardless of the drug chosen, the involuntary contractions of the bladder are not abolished and the degree of improvement is modest.
- Many of the drugs have side-effects.
- Many of the drugs are costly.

- Drugs should only be used in conjunction with other therapy, e.g. behavioural approaches, and only after other factors contributing to incontinence have been addressed.
- The choice of drug should be based on individual requirements, taking account of the side-effects, half-life and onset of action of the drug.
- Regardless of the drug chosen, the initial dose should be relatively low and increased slowly to balance efficacy against side-effects.
- Patients must be monitored for urinary retention.

Drugs used for stress incontinence

The high concentration of alpha-adrenergic receptors in the bladder neck, bladder base and proximal urethra may be stimulated by alpha-adrenergic agonists, with resultant contraction and bladder outlet resistance. This is useful in patients with urethral insufficiency causing stress incontinence. Other drugs that will enhance the alpha-adrenergic response will also increase bladder outlet resistance. The drugs used in the treatment of stress incontinence therefore fall into three main categories.

Alpha-adrenergic agonist agents. The drug phenylpropanolamine in sustained release form is the main drug of this type used in women with stress incontinence (AHCPR, 1992). Eight randomised controlled trials were reviewed by the panel (AHCPR, 1992), and no newer studies have since been found. There were varying responses to therapy, and side-effects were minimal. It was concluded that therapy using phenylpropanolamine appears to produce few cures but may subjectively improve 30–60% of patients over placebo response. Its use in women with hypertension required further investigation.

Oestrogen therapy. This is considered useful in postmenopausal women as it may increase proliferation of urethral mucosa and increase vascularity, tone and the responsiveness of the urethral muscle to alpha-adrenergic agents. Oestrogen therapy has been prescribed orally and vaginally, and for patients with stress and urge incontinence (AHCPR, 1992). Cardozo and Kelleher (1994) noted that studies have varied with the type of oestrogen, route of administration and dose and duration of therapy used.

Fantl *et al.* (1994) undertook a meta-analysis of studies testing the effectiveness of oestrogen therapy in postmenopausal women with urinary incontinence. They found that 143 out of 166 articles published between 1969 and 1992 did not meet their criteria for inclusion in their review. There were only six controlled and seventeen uncontrolled trials. The meta-analysis showed that oestrogen therapy significantly improves urinary incontinence subjectively. However, objective improvement could not be confirmed as there was no significant effect on urine loss and the significant effects on maximum urethral closure pressure could have been accounted for by one study showing a large effect. The meta-analysis is weakened, however, since it involved studies that included non-homogenous groups and which varied considerably with regard to therapeutic interventions used, diagnostic criteria and outcome measures.

Cardozo and Kelleher (1994) and Fantl et al. (1994) concluded that the subjective benefits of oestrogen therapy might be due to the effect of oestrogen on other organs, enhancing the overall quality of life of the individual.

Combined alpha-adrenergic agonist and oestrogen supplement therapy. By combining these two types of therapy, the number and/or sensitivity of alpha-adrenergic receptors in the urethra are increased, thus enhancing the effects of alpha-adrenergic agonists. Only four randomised controlled trials were identified by the AHCPR guideline which had shown that combined therapy might be more beneficial than alpha-adrenergic agonists alone (AHCPR, 1992). A further study by Ahlstrom et al. (1990) involved 29 postmenopausal women with stress incontinence and oestrogen deficiency in a randomised, double blind cross-over trial of oestriol plus phenylpropanolamine and oestriol plus placebo. Combined treatment was found significantly to improve leakage episodes, whereas oestriol alone did not. Both treatments produced significant subjective improvements in incontinence. Ahlstrom et al. (1990) concluded that combined treatment was more effective than oestriol alone for stress incontinence. The AHCPR (1992) suggested that combination therapy be used when the initial single therapy fails.

Other drugs. The AHCPR guideline made reference to two other drugs used for stress incontinence. Imipramine has been reported to benefit women with stress incontinence, although no controlled studies are available to substantiate this evidence. Propranolol, a beta-adrenergic blocking drug, was not recommended by the AHCPR because of the limited evidence of its effects (AHCPR, 1992).

Drugs used for nocturnal enuresis

In addition to the use of imipramine described earlier, desmopressin acetate (DDAVP) is also often recommended for nocturnal enuresis. This drug, a vasopressin analogue with anti-diuretic properties, has become widely used for both children and adults.

Moffat *et al.* (1993) undertook a systematic review of all RCTs using DDAVP to treat nocturnal enuresis for all age groups. Articles published in English, indexed on MEDLINE and published between 1962 and 1992 were searched. Only 18 articles, referred to true randomised controlled trials. Moffat *et al.* (1993) concluded that these studies demonstrated that DDAVP was effective in reducing the number of wet nights in children for whom other treatments had failed. However, it produces complete dryness in only a minority, and this is often a temporary effect. Side-effects were reported as minor and infrequent, including headaches, abdominal pain, nasal stuffiness and epistaxis, the latter possibly related to the use of the drug in a nasal spray. There were insufficient long-term studies identified in the review by Moffat *et al.* (1993) to determine the long-term efficacy of DDAVP. In comparison with other therapies, Moffat *et al.* (1993) concluded that DDAVP was inferior to conditioning alarms as a primary therapy.

Summary

Drug therapy is therefore recommended in some circumstances for detrusor instability, nocturnal enuresis and stress incontinence. However, in almost all cases, the evidence for the use of these drugs is *not* based on adequate research data from randomised controlled trials.

Management of incontinence

The aim of care and treatment of the person suffering from incontinence is the return to continence. However, when a return to full continence has not been achieved, social continence is the goal. This can be achieved through the use of various aids and appliances to manage the incontinence. These are grouped into three main categories: containment aids, conduction aids and occlusive devices (Ryan-Wooley, 1987). The literature concerning these three categories is considered and areas of consensus highlighted.

Containment aids

Two excellent reviews of the research studies undertaken on the various types of containment aid were found (Brink, 1990; Cottenden, 1992), which gave an overview of the issues involved. Two types of containment aid exist: body-worn pads/pants and underpads, which are used to protect chairs and beds. These may each be either reusable or disposable. There are a wide variety of each of these types available and the *Directory of Aids and Appliances*, published by ACA (1988), provides information on those available in the United Kingdom. A revised directory is to be published by the Continence Foundation in 1998.

The reviews by Brink (1990) and Cottenden (1992) described and critiqued many studies comparing different products. However, both concluded that there is little point in comparisons being made between specific products since there are so many different products available, with a rapid turnover and change in technical specifications of products as well as limited criteria against which to make judgements. Cottenden and Ledger (1993) reported on an international multicentre study that developed accurate laboratory tests for determining the leakage performance of incontinence pads. This work will be used to enable the determination of international standards for testing absorbent products and should facilitate future research. Philp *et al.* (1993) described the key features for absorbent body-worn pads but it is not clear how these were derived and whether or not they are research-based.

Further studies have been identified comparing various products (Hanley, 1992; Gibb and Wong, 1994), including studies of reusable products (Philp *et al.*, 1992; Norris *et al.*, 1993) and underpads (Thornburn *et al.*, 1992). A study by Hellstrom *et al.* (1993) that adapted incontinence aids to patients' leakage volumes, as determined by pad weighing tests and a severity index, was also reviewed. This study concluded that aids should be prescribed according to individual need. However, McKeever (1990), in a study of recognised incontinence, found a large proportion of patients who had been prescribed pads without a prior assessment. The conclusions drawn from these studies regarding particular products are not very useful for the reasons already given. There is, however, a consensus between the overall conclusions of these studies and the reviews of Brink (1990) and Cottenden (1992); these provide a useful overview of the issues of good practice regarding the use of containment aids for urinary incontinence and are therefore summarised below:

- Absorbent products should not be prescribed until a thorough assessment has been undertaken of individuals, their incontinence, abilities and disabilities, their lifestyle and environment and that of their carers where appropriate.
- Absorbent products may be helpful in conjunction with other therapy and should not be the first line of management.
- Products issued must meet the needs of the individual.
- Patient choice and the subjective impression of a product are important.
- A wide range of sizes and absorbencies should be available from which to select for a patient. Selecting the correct size and absorbency can aid comfort and security.
- Careful instructions should be given to users of the products by both manufacturers and health care professionals.
- Individuals should be reassessed regularly as their needs are likely to change with time.
- Future research should be collaborative, both between health care professionals and manufacturers and between a network of centres prepared to trial products.
- Future research should involve larger clinical trials and should be designed to focus on classes of product rather than specific products, as the latter change so regularly and are so numerous.

Conduction aids

Three categories of conduction appliance exist: male appliances, female appliances and catheters. Each will be discussed.

Male collection appliances

Body-worn urinals comprise a semi-rigid rubber cone that is held in place over the penis by belts and straps and is connected to a drainage bag. A pubic pressure flange may also be attached for use with men with retracted penises. There was no published research on the use of body-worn urinals or pubic pressure flanges. These aids should fitted by an experienced appliance fitter, and the wearer needs sufficient manual dexterity to manage them. A high standard of personal hygiene is required with their use. Wearers have complained of bulkiness, soreness and sweatiness (Cottenden, 1992).

Penile sheaths act as collecting devices and are attached to urine drainage bags. Cottenden (1992) reviewed the limited research relating to the use of these appliances, and no further research has been found. Conclusions drawn from the review by Cottenden (1992) and the AHCPR (1992) guideline are that:

- Penile sheaths may be useful for short-term use.
- Penile sheaths should not be used for anyone with outflow obstruction, symptomatic urinary tract infection or a retracted penis.
- Allergic reactions, skin rashes and erythema may be associated with the use of penile sheaths.
- Penile sheaths are associated with urinary tract infections.
- Hygiene is important, and sheaths should be changed at least daily to relieve pressure and allow inspection of the skin.

Female conduction appliances

Female conduction appliances are available but have not been used to any great extent. Adverse reactions to the devices include periurethral erythema and perineal itching (Cottenden, 1992). Pieper and Cleland (1993) have reported on a new female collecting device, but its efficacy has yet to be adequately demonstrated.

Catheters

Indwelling urethral catheter. Catheterisation is usually considered as a last resort in the management of incontinence, and indwelling catheters are only used when other techniques have failed. The period of time for which a patient is catheterised can vary from a few days (short term) to a number of years (long term), the latter being especially the case in incontinence sufferers. In one health district, 4% of patients known to the district nursing service were using a long-term catheter. Problems associated with indwelling catheters are infection, leakage, pain, encrustation and blockage (Roe, 1992a). Catheter care and urinary tract infection associated with catheterisation have been widely researched, research which is discussed in excellent reviews by Roe (1992c, 1993) and Gould (1994). The following areas of consensus regarding indwelling catheter care were synthesised from these reviews:

- Indwelling catheters should only be used out of medical necessity of when it is the patient's choice.
- There is a great risk of urinary tract infection associated with indwelling catheters, and bacteriuria has shown to be inevitable

within 3–4 weeks. Catheter-associated urinary tract infection can increase mortality.

- For the general drainage of free-flowing urine, small charrière (12–16 Ch) catheters and small balloons should be used. Pain and leakage have been found to be associated with large balloons.
- Catheter surfaces and balloons exposed to urine will develop encrustations. Encrustation occurs in all types of catheter. Long-term catheters are significantly more likely to suffer recurrent encrustations and subsequent blockage than are short-term ones. The use of mini bladder washouts with the weak citric acid solution of magnesium oxide (Suby G) may be effective in treating and preventing encrustation, but this requires further research evidence before it can be recommended (Getliffe, 1994).
- Research evidence on effective meatal care is lacking. From the evidence that is currently available, it is known that meatal care is best achieved through thorough attention to personal hygiene, using soap and water and clean wash-cloths.
- Research evidence on the benefits of catheter clamping for long-term catheter patients is limited. There was no research evidence on the use of catheter valves, which have recently become popular and which allow the bladder to fill and urine to be drained intermittently.
- Drainage bag selection is dependent upon the reasons for catheterisation, the duration of use, patient choice and factors relating to the prevention of cross-infection.
- Emptying and changing the drainage bag constitutes a potential break in the closed system, and a clean technique for emptying the bag should be taught to avoid cross-infection.
- In order to prevent nosocomial infection in hospital, used drainage bags must be disposed of. Until further research is undertaken on the reuse or disposal of drainage bags in the community, patients may choose to dispose of their bags or reuse the drainage bags after washing them through with soap and hot water and allowing them to dry thoroughly.
- Reusable leg drainage bags have been employed in one case series without an increase in urinary tract infection attributable to the use of such bags (Rooney, 1994). Further evidence from controlled trials is required to demonstrate their safety.
- There should be a continual review of the necessity for the catheter.

Suprapubic catheterisation. This involves the percutaneous or surgical introduction of a catheter into the bladder via the abdominal wall. The use of suprapubic catheters for the management of incontinence has been limited but has recently grown, their use being generally short term following gynaecological, urological and other types of surgery. However, they can be used long term in men and women, particularly for bladder obstruction as an alternative to urethral catheterisation. The suprapubic catheter may be a preferred alternative to urethral catheterisation in sexually active adults as the latter may in some cases inhibit sexual function. Immediate complications may be associated with the introduction of the catheter, e.g. bowel injury and haematoma, or with local effects of urine on the skin. Long-term complications are reported to be similar to those of urethral catheterisation (AHCPR, 1992).

Horgan *et al.* (1992) undertook a follow-up study for 3 years of 86 patients admitted to an accident and emergency unit with acute retention of urine resulting from enlargement of the prostate gland. Fifty-six were catheterised suprapubically and 30 urethrally. The men catheterised suprapubically suffered less urinary tract infection, urethral stricture and epididymo-orchitis than did those catheterised urethrally, although those with suprapubic catheters experienced more frequent dislodgement of the catheter. However, no statistical analysis was performed, and this was not a randomised controlled trial.

Vandoni *et al.* (1994) found, in a random prospective trial of 50 patients, that those with suprapubic catheters experienced significantly less bacteriuria than did those with urethral catheters. There were no significant differences between the two groups in terms of the pain and discomfort experienced.

Apart from this, there is very little research related to this form of management for incontinence. The AHCPR (1992) panel concluded that a suprapubic catheter would be preferable to an indwelling urethral catheter in the male who requires chronic bladder drainage and for whom no other form of management is possible. They caution, however, that this would require the education of health care professionals in the management of such catheters.

Intermittent catheterisation. The technique of clean intermittent catheterisation has been shown to be a safe and effective way of managing a patient with a neurogenic bladder and/or overflow incontinence for over 20 years (Winder, 1992; Oakeshott and Hunt, 1992). The technique has been used with patients of all ages and both sexes, and even by highly disabled individuals (Bakke *et al.*, 1992; Lin-Dyken *et al.*, 1992). Clean intermittent catheterisation is associated with lower rates of urinary tract infection (Winder, 1992) and fewer complications to the upper urinary tract and renal function than the use of indwelling catheters (Lin-Dyken *et al.*, 1992; Oakeshott and Hunt, 1992). Patients are afforded more control over their incontinence with this technique (Oakeshott and Hunt, 1992), and the majority of patients using clean intermittent catheterisation in Norway during 1988 considered the technique to be an advantage, were not averse to the procedure and found it easy to perform (Bakke *et al.*, 1993).

An interview study of 26 randomly chosen teenagers and young adults with myelomeningocele who had been using the procedure for 7.5–12 years found that clean intermittent catheterisation was a well-accepted part of life. No one in the group wanted to return to the previous voiding technique. However, careful introduction, continuous support and consistent encouragement were necessary to maintain these results (Lindehall *et al.*, 1994).

Winder (1992) explains the technique and the required patient teaching involved. She stresses that patients must be motivated, have the relevant manual dexterity and be taught by an adequately prepared health care professional.

Occlusive and other devices

Occlusive devices such as penile clamps are available but are rarely used. Clamps must be removed at 3-hourly intervals to empty the bladder. Complications associated with their incorrect use include urethral erosion, penile oedema, pain and obstruction. There were no research studies related to their use (AHCPR, 1992).

Pessaries designed to reduce pelvic prolapse and alleviate the symptoms of pelvic relaxation have been used for incontinence but without evidence of their efficacy (AHCPR, 1992). A bladderneck support prosthesis was evaluated in 32 physically active women (mean age 46) with stress incontinence, using both objective and subjective outcome measurements. Significant improvements in both outcome measurements were found, and 83% women were dry with the device in place. The subjects found the device to be comfortable (Davila and Ostermann, 1994). However, more studies and clinical trials are needed to confirm these results.

Summary

There are a variety of approaches to the management of incontinence, and the research evidence on the efficacy of these has been found to be variable. Regardless of the approach or appliance chosen, there was consensus on the following four principles:

1. All patients must be carefully assessed by an adequately trained health care professional before any strategy for the management of incontinence is implemented. No aid or appliance should be issued without such an assessment.
2. The promotion of continence should be the aim for all patients. The management of incontinence should occur concurrently with strategies for the promotion of continence, or only when such strategies have been shown to fail.
3. Patient choice should be a key consideration in the determination of management approach and selection of aids.
4. All patients should be regularly reviewed, as their needs are likely to change and the management approach will, therefore, also need to change.

Faecal incontinence

The research basis of the aetiology, assessment and management of faecal incontinence has been the subject of several excellent recent reviews (Barrett, 1992, 1993; Hallan et al., 1993; Jorge and Wexner, 1993; Bartolo et al., 1994). Barrett (1992, 1993) provides a good review of the literature and focuses particularly on the medical management of faecal incontinence in elderly people. Since this is the group in which prevalence is greatest and they are most likely to present to GPs, this review is recommended. Hallan et al. (1993), Jorge and Wexner (1993) and Bartolo et al. (1994) reviewed the literature and provide useful information on the various surgical options for treatment. Jorge and Wexner (1993) included a tabulation of the results of studies of various surgical techniques. Felt-Bersma and Cuesta (1994) outline the various tests and treatments that may be use. The use of biofeedback as an approach to the management of faecal incontinence is reviewed in two papers (Enck, 1993; Bassotti and Whitehead, 1994) and by Barrett (1993).

The following summary of consensus opinion on faecal incontinence of relevance to the primary health care team is synthesised from these reviews.

The problem of faecal incontinence has been shown to affect all ages, including children, but is most common in the elderly. Studies of the prevalence of faecal incontinence in the community suggest that fewer than 4 people per 1000 of the population aged 15–64 years suffer from the condition but that this figure rises after the age of 65 to 11 per 1000 for men and 13.3 per 1000 for women (Thomas *et al.*, 1984). Faecal incontinence is more common in elderly people in institutional care (Barrett, 1993). Sufferers may have had symptoms for years before seeking help, and many may have disguised the complaint as 'diarrhoea'. The social and psychological effects of faecal incontinence on individuals and their carers can be quite marked (Smith and Smith, 1993).

Faecal incontinence is caused by:

• colorectal disease/diarrhoea;
• anorectal incontinence (idiopathic incontinence) due to weaknesses of the external and/or internal anal sphincters and pelvic floor muscles, possibly caused by childbirth (Swash, 1993), anorectal surgery, trauma, fistulae and abscesses, or the effects of ageing, although a combination of these is often involved;
• faecal impaction, the most common cause in elderly people, although retention of faeces in children is also a common cause of faecal incontinence;
• neurological causes including neurological disease involving the pelvic floor and the central nervous system, dementia, unconsciousness and behavioural causes;
• developmental causes, e.g. in individuals with learning difficulties.

Other contributory factors that may predispose an individual to faecal incontinence and/or exacerbate an existing condition include:

1. fluid and dietary intake, especially fibre intake–either too much or too little;
2. the inappropriate use of laxatives;
3. medications;
4. inappropriate toileting habits and toilet training in children;
5. immobility;
6. other physical disability, e.g. arthritis.

Very often, several of these causes and factors are involved.

Assessment of the patient should comprise a full medical history, including the history of the incontinence, defaecation history, fluid

and dietary intake, medications, and neurological, surgical, gynaecological and obstetric history. Physical examination should include the
assessment of mobility and general functioning, neurological assessment, abdominal palpation and rectal examination, and examination of the perineum.

Additional tests that may be required include abdominal X-ray,
full blood count, faecal occult bloods, thyroid function tests and
specific bowel investigations such as sigmoidoscopy, barium enema
and colonoscopy if colorectal disease is suspected. Patients may be
referred for anorectal function tests. There were no clear guidelines
in the literature regarding criteria to determine when a patient
should be referred by the GP and which additional tests should be
undertaken by whom.

Treatment of faecal incontinence is related to the cause. A diagnosis of the cause is therefore required.

In cases of faecal impaction, the aim is to clear the bowel of
faeces and then prevent the recurrence of constipation by keeping
the bowel empty. This may be achieved through the initial use of
enemas and then laxatives. The choice of laxative should be determined by the character of the stool and the person's ability to
defaecate.

Antidiarrhoeal drugs such as loperamide may be used to alter
stool consistency when diarrhoea is a cause of incontinence while
other causes are investigated.

Biofeedback has been used successfully in patients with anorectal
incontinence, although the definitive mode of action remains
unclear.

Electrical stimulation has achieved varied results in patients with
faecal incontinence (Barrett, 1992; Scheuer et al., 1994).

Various surgical options for treatment are available for anorectal
incontinence with reported reasonable success rates, although they
have not been subjected to randomised controlled trials.

Faecal incontinence in the elderly can usually be successfully
treated by simple conservative measures, with complete restoration
of faecal continence in over 80% of cases.

Educational issues

Several issues have been raised by this review of the literature in relation to the education of the public, the patient and health care
professionals. These will be considered here with suggestions for
improvements where necessary.

Education and the general public

This review has shown that urinary incontinence is a common problem, affecting between 2% and 10% of men and 8% and 25% of women. Prevalence studies of urinary incontinence in the United Kingdom revealed that between 12% and 50% of people with urinary incontinence did not consult their doctors about their complaint (Jolleys, 1988; O'Brien et al., 1991; Brocklehurst, 1993; Harrison and Memel, 1994). These and other studies have also shown that people are in fact reluctant to tell anyone about their problem.

Reymert and Hunskaar (1994) found that 36% of the perimenopausal women in their study had told no one and 28% had told only their husbands or a friend. The most common reason given in all these studies for not seeking help was because the incontinence was not a problem for the person. However, the next most frequently given reasons relate more to the public's lack of understanding of the condition. People thought that urinary incontinence was 'normal for their age' and 'a usual female complaint', and that 'no help was available' and 'nothing could be done' (Jolleys, 1988; Goldstein et al., 1992; Harrison and Memel, 1994; Reymert and Hunskaar, 1994). This review of urinary incontinence has shown that all these assumptions by the general public are in fact false and that urinary incontinence can be treated and often cured in the majority of cases.

However, some studies have shown that a minority of people did not come forward for help because of embarrassment (Jolleys, 1988; Goldstein et al., 1992; Reymert and Hunskaar, 1994) and that of those who did come forward, some were nonetheless embarrassed when talking to their doctors (Brocklehurst, 1993). It was interesting to note that in Jolleys' (1988) survey of patients from her own practice, 166 out of the 343 women who reported suffering incontinence did not even answer the question 'Why have you not spoken to the doctor about your incontinence?'. One possible reason for this may be reluctance on the part of the women to even admit to their embarrassment or ignorance, a factor proposed by Reymert and Hunskaar (1994) in their study. They suggest that women may be embarrassed about their embarrassment and therefore reluctant to disclose their actual feelings about the urinary incontinence. The effects of urinary incontinence on individuals have been discussed earlier in this review, and the stigma that can be associated with the condition has been highlighted.

It is therefore evident that the educational issues concerning the public are twofold. First, there is a need for the public to be given facts about incontinence, its causes and treatment, as well as preventive health care measures. Second, the stigma and embarrassment associated with the condition must be removed. The latter may happen automatically once the public are aware of the facts surrounding the condition, and therefore both issues are linked.

Attempts have been made to tackle the issue of public education by the Department of Health through the 'Continence Awareness' week in 1994 and the 'Dry day, dry night' awareness campaign in 1995. Incontinence advisory telephone services have been provided in several areas (Brown and White, 1991; Dawes, 1994) and have reported large numbers of enquirers. Other attempts to make advice and treatment more easily accessible have been the provision of open access continence clinics (Morrison *et al.*, 1992; Brown, 1994), although Harrison and Memel (1994) found that a health promotion clinic did not prove to be an efficient setting in which to offer continence services.

Patient education

In addition to the need to educate the general public, there is a need to educate patients and/or their carers about the promotion and management of continence for their own condition. This literature review has demonstrated how the motivation and positive participation of the patient is a key issue in the success of promotion strategies such as pelvic floor exercises and bladder training, and in the use of intermittent self-catheterisation as a management approach. Roe (1992b) discussed the research related to patient education with particular reference to continence care. The health care professional must be aware of the need to teach the patient effectively if the promotion and management of continence is to be successful.

Education of health care professionals

Evidence that there is a need for further education of health care professionals comes from a variety of sources in this country as well as studies from abroad (Sandvik *et al.*, 1990). Brocklehurst (1993) found that fewer than 25% of patients with urinary incontinence were given a full examination by their GPs. Amongst those patients in the study by O'Brien *et al.* (1991) who had discussed their problem with their GP or a nurse, only 20% had been assessed in the previous year and 30% reported never having had an assessment.

Oakeshott and Hunt (1992) referred to a survey of 55 GPs of whom 29, including four lecturers in general practice, indicated that they did not know anything about intermittent self-catheterisation. Deficits in the knowledge of GPs about urinary incontinence were found by Jolleys and Wilson (1993) in a survey of 1284 GPs. They also found that GPs lacked confidence in their abilities to diagnose and manage urinary incontinence, although this lack of confidence was not related to length of practice as a GP.

GPs could refer patients to continence advisers, who have specialist knowledge and expertise (Rhodes and Parker, 1993). However, Briggs and Williams (1992) found that 42 out of 101 GPs surveyed never used the services of continence advisers for older patients.

In her study of nurses' attitudes to incontinence, Cheater (1991a) found that there was a need for the increased education of nurses in relation to preventative care and the therapeutic and rehabilitation aspects of continence promotion. Cheater (1992) also found that qualified nurses lacked the knowledge to complete an adequate assessment of incontinent patients. Health visitors wanted more information on enuresis in a training needs analysis by Burnet et al. (1992). The need for social service staff to receive in-service education on continence promotion and for the topic to be included in NVQ modules for care assistants was highlighted by Swaffield (1994).

The paucity of education on incontinence in medical education is identified by Brocklehurst (1990b), who stated that an average of 70 minutes was devoted to urinary incontinence and 20 minutes to faecal incontinence in undergraduate courses. A hospital doctors survey on urinary incontinence was undertaken in 1994 by the Training Committee of the British Geriatrics Society for Health in Old Age. It concluded that almost two-thirds of senior registrars were not receiving exposure to specialist training in the management of continence (i.e. attachment to a geriatrician with a special interest in incontinence management or other specialist who provided special clinics or investigation units and participation in research in urinary incontinence). It also found that training programmes varied between regions (Lynham, 1994, personal communication).

The necessity for the further and improved education of health care professionals is therefore apparent, and Rhodes (1994) argues that continence advisers are best placed to provide this, although this need not always be through formal teaching sessions.

Szonyi and Millard (1994) undertook a controlled trial of an education package on urinary incontinence for GPs in New South

Wales, Australia. They had a very poor response to their initial questionnaire requesting participants to join the study, only 16.3% of the 510 GPs replying. Those GPs who completed the education package showed a significant improvement in their knowledge compared with those who did not use the package. Their increase in knowledge related only to those areas covered by the package, and there is therefore no way of knowing whether or not the GPs had used the package directly to answer the questions on the post-test or whether this represented a genuine increase in their knowledge.

Summary

This review has demonstrated the need for education of the public, patient/carer and professional. Despite some recent efforts, all three areas remain to be adequately addressed by the health service and require attention since education is the key to the successful promotion and management of continence.

Audit issues

There is no research in the literature regarding the auditing specifically of continence services in the community, although the CARE Scheme by the Royal College of Physicians, involving a clinical audit of the long-term care of elderly people, included questionnaires for audit of urinary and faecal incontinence (RCP, 1992). Guidelines for purchasers produced by West Midlands Regional Health Authority (Brocklehurst, 1994) and the Continence Foundation (1995) provided information on auditing. Corbett-Nolan (1994) described how one regional health authority set up a working group to determine standards for continence advisory services.

It is essential that services for the promotion and management of continence are audited regularly. Brocklehurst (1994) recommends that purchasers, which includes fundholding GPs identify groups whose continence needs have been identified as rarely being met, including children, those with disabilities and people from ethnic minorities. He recommends that information on service provision to these particular groups should be provided in annual and quarterly reviews. Record-keeping systems should allow health care professionals to identify patients who report incontinence as a symptom or sign and not only those in whom it is a diagnosis. Various outcome measures can be used to audit the continence service provided by the PHCT, which should include consumer views on the service (Brocklehurst, 1994).

Conclusion

This systematic review of the literature has considered the prevalence and incidence of urinary incontinence. The burden of the
condition was described in terms of costs to the health service and
the individual as well as of the personal burden of the sufferer.
Causes and types of urinary incontinence were outlined. The assessment of a patient presenting with urinary incontinence (including
enuresis) was specified, and issues surrounding the need for urodynamic evaluation were analysed. The research basis of strategies for
the promotion and management of urinary continence was considered and recommendations for practice were given. Faecal incontinence was discussed briefly, and reference was made to recent
reviews of relevant literature. Finally, the educational and audit
issues were examined and recommendations made.

This systematic review has clearly identified the areas of consensus that exist within the published literature on the promotion and
management of continence as well as highlighting those aspects
which require further research.

Chapter 5
Recommendations for further research and development

The following areas were identified through review of the literature and during the consensus conference as requiring further research and development, to improve both the evidence supporting clinical practice and clinical practice itself. They relate to the promotion of continence and management of incontinence in all settings and not only for the PHCT.

- Any research undertaken should utilise standardised definitions and approaches in order to increase the comparability of studies and the opportunities for meta-analysis.
- An epidemiological study of normal voiding and defaecation in children is required in order to increase the understanding of enuresis and encopresis.
- The type and effectiveness of the current provision of care by the PHCT, including school nurses and community medical officers, for children with enuresis and encopresis is largely unknown at present, and there is therefore a need for further research in this area.
- Further research is required to identify the causes and risk factors related to urinary and faecal incontinence, thereby increasing the possibilities of prevention. This should include:
  - incidence studies of urinary and faecal incontinence;
  - studies of the physiology of the anorectum;
  - randomised controlled trials on the relationship between labour, episiotomy and faecal incontinence.

- Whilst there is an emerging body of knowledge on the impact of incontinence on the quality of life of individuals, further research is required, particularly in relation to faecal incontinence.
- Research to establish the reliability and validity of assessment tools is necessary.
- Further research, in the form of randomised controlled trials, is required to test the long-term efficacy of bladder training, pelvic floor exercises, vaginal cones, electrical stimulation and biofeedback, to determine effective treatment patterns and the motivational support required.
- Multicentre randomised controlled trials of drug therapies and surgical techniques for incontinence are required in order for clinicians to make informed decisions regarding care.
- There is a need for the development of a drug that would treat internal anal sphincter weakness without causing constipation, thus reducing the need for surgery.
- The development of pelvic floor surgery as a specialism treating both urinary and faecal incontinence should be considered.
- Independent, multicentre, randomised controlled trials using preset standardised criteria are necessary to test the efficacy of the various main types of aid and appliance available.
- There should be greater multidisciplinary education of all health care professionals at preregistration level to increase the awareness of continence promotion.
- There should be increased specialist training provided on the promotion of continence and the management of incontinence at postregistration level for all GPs, nurses and other health care professionals.

Appendix I
Examples of good practice and/or useful resources

Reference	Abstract
Addison R, Roe B, Taylor P (1994) The Role of the Continence Advisor. Clinical Practice–A Principal Function. London: RCN.	A report of workshops that considered one of the few principle functions of the continence adviser–clinical practice– and established consensus standards of care relating to types of incontinence. The methodology used is presented along with the consensus standards of care.
AHCPR (1992) Urinary Incontinence in Adults: Clinical Practice Guideline. Rockville, MD: US Department of Health and Human Sciences, Agency for Health Care Policy and Research.	This consensus guideline aims to improve the reporting, diagnosis and treatment of urinary incontinence, reduce variations in clinical practice and educate health profes sionals and consumers about the condition. It applies to acquired urinary incontinence in adults does not apply to children. Extraurethral urinary incontinence is not addressed.
Association for Continence Advice (1988) Directory of Continence and Toileting Aids. London: Disabled Living Foundation.	This is a very useful resource that outlines products available for the management of incontinence and relevant supplies and manufacturers. An updated version is to be published by the Continence Foundation in 1998.
Association for Continence Advice (1993) Guidelines for Continence Care. London: ACA.	These guidelines are to indicate what clients should expect from health services, local authorities, employers and those offering public services in order to manage continence problems. They also aim to guide providers of services, raising awareness of the facilities required. These are clearly written and provide a useful guide to continence services provision, but direct guidelines for practice lack reference to supporting research.

(contd)

Reference	Abstract
Barrett JA (1993) Faecal Incontinence and Related Problems in the Older Adult. London: Edward Arnold.	A useful textbook that specifically addresses faecal incontinence, including the physiological aspects and practical management of this condition. The book is based on recent research and is very well referenced.
Brocklehurst N (1994) Purchasing for Continence Promotion. Guidelines for Health Authorities and GP Fundholders or Commissioning Continence Services. West Midlands Regional Health Authority.	A very useful booklet that is designed to help purchasers develop effective conti- nence services. It is well written, referenced and provides examples of good practice.
Butler RJ (1993) Enuresis Resource Pack. Bristol: ERIC.	This pack contains charts, question- naires and information to assist health care professionals dealing with children with enuresis.
Charter for Continence (1995) Developed by The Continence Foundation, InContact, ACA, RCN Continence Care Forum, ERIC, Spinal Injuries Association and Multiple Sclerosis Society. Produced by an educational grant from Bard Limited.	This Charter presents the specific needs and rights of people with bladder or bowel problems. It outlines the resources available and the standards of care that can be expected. It is available in nine different languages: English, Cantonese, Welsh, Somali, Hindi, Urdu, Punjabi, Bengali and Gujarati. Copies, including posters, are available from: Bard Limited, Forest House, Brighton Road, Crawley, West Sussex RH11 9BP. Tel: (01293) 527888; or from the Continence Foundation on 0171–404 6875.
Clark G, Fleming C, Habel A *et al.* (1994) Nocturnal Enuresis: A Strategy for Management. Hospital Update, September, Supplement. Produced in conjunction with Ferring Pharmaceuticals Ltd.	This report of a working party provides protocols for clinical assessment and age-related management plans for nocturnal enuresis.
Continence Foundation (1992) Continence in Primary Care–A Resource Pack. London: Continence Foundation.	This resource pack was originally designed and developed in Australia and was adapted for use in the United Kingdom by the Continence Foundation and distributed in 1992. It contains several useful leaflets, protocols and reference material.

Reference	Abstract
Continence Foundation (1994) The Continence Guide '94. London: Continence Foundation.	This booklet was written for individuals who suffer from bowel or bladder problems and provides easy-to-read practical advice and explanations. A very useful resource for sufferers and their carers.
Continence Foundation (1995) Guidelines on Working with Ethnic Minority Committees. London: Continence Foundation.	A useful, brief document outlining issues to consider when working with ethnic minority communities.
ERIC (1995) Charter for Children with Bedwetting and Daytime Wetting and Their Families. Bristol: ERIC.	This Charter presents the specific needs and rights of children who experience bedwetting and daytime wetting and guidance for their families. It outlines the resources available and standards of care that can be expected. Copies are available from ERIC.
Morgan R (1993) Guidelines on Minimum Standards of Practice in the Treatment of Enuresis. Bristol: ERIC.	These guidelines are in the form of minimum standards for an enuresis service. Target standards are also given that enable the improvement of existing services. Referral, assessment, treatment and evaluation are covered. There are few references to support recommendations for practice, but this document is a very useful guide for purchasers and providers to the service levels required.
NHS Executive (1995) Incontinence–Patients' Perceptions of Services. Leeds: NHS Executive.	This booklet is part of a series aimed primarily at purchasers. It represents the views of users of continence services, although no details are given of how these were derived. It poses challenges to purchasers of services and is a useful reminder of the relevance of consumers' views.
RCP (1995) Incontinence: Causes, Management and Provision of Services. A Report of the Royal College of Physicians. London: RCP.	A report produced by a working party of the Royal College of Physicians. It covers both urinary and faecal incontinence and is intended as a guide for health professionals as well as purchasers and providers.

(contd)

Reference	Abstract
Rhodes P, Parker G (1993) The Role of Continence Advisers in England and Wales. University of York: SPRU.	The report of a research study into the role of continence advisers. It provides useful information on the history and changing role of the continence advisor and considers the implications for future continence services.
Roe BH (ed.) (1992) Clinical Nursing Practice. The Promotion and Management of Continence. London: Prentice Hall.	This edited book provides an excellent review of the research evidence for the promotion and management of urinary and faecal continence. It is well written and very well referenced. A useful resource for all health professionals.
Roe B, Addison RR, Clayton J (1992) The Role of the Continence Advisor. London: RCN.	Report of consensus workshops held by RCN Continence Care for UK. A mission statement and four principal functions of continence advisors are identified and discussed.
Roe B, Williams K (1994) Clinical Handbook for Continence Care. London: Scutari Press.	This is a useful practical handbook with research-based recommendations for clinical practice.
SE Thames RHA (1994) Standards for Continence Advisory Services. Report from a Working Group of the SE Thames Continence Advisers Group. Bexhill on Sea: SETRHA.	This report of a working group identifies standards for continence services and is aimed at commissioners, providers and users of accrediting services. These are not based on research evidence.
Smith N, Clamp M (1991) Continence Promotion in General Practice. Oxford: Oxford University Press.	A practical guide to incontinence for the GP, it is clearly written and focuses on treatments available to the GP. However, it has few supporting references.

Appendix II
Useful addresses

Association for Continence Advice
2 Doughty Street
London WC1N 2PH
0171–404 6821

British Digestive Foundation
3 St Andrew's Place
London NW1 4LB

Charter for Continence
Copies available from:
Bard Ltd
Forest House
Brighton Road
Crawley
West Sussex RH11 9BP
(01293) 527888

Continence Foundation
2 Doughty Street
London WC1N 2PH
0171–404 6875 (Tel)
0171–404 6876 (Fax)

Enuresis Resource and Information Centre (ERIC)
65 St Michael's Hill
Bristol BS2 8DZ
0117–926 4920

InContact
(National Action on Incontinence)
The Basement
2 Doughty Street
London WC1N 2PH

Incontinence Information Helpline (run by the Continence
Foundation)
0191–213 0050

Appendix III
Methodology

Introduction

These guidelines were commissioned in 1994 by the NHS Executive as part of their Consensus Strategy for Major Clinical Guidelines. The project objectives were originally as follows:

1. To undertake a critical review of published literature relating to incontinence.
2. To develop guidelines for the promotion and management of continence for use by members of the PHCT.
3. To obtain consensus on the guidelines for the promotion and management of continence from a conference of invited experts in the field of incontinence.
4. To implement the guidelines for the promotion and management of continence with members of the PHCT in one general practice.
5. To evaluate the clinical impact of the guidelines on the promotion and management of continence.

After discussion with the Strategy Director, Professor Michael Deighan, it was decided to develop the guidelines after, rather than before, the conference.

Management arrangements

A Steering Group for the project was formed, and a Project Officer appointed. An expert panel of delegates for the conference was determined, ensuring adequate representation from the different relevant professions, professional organisations and consumer groups. The guidelines were intended for use by the PHCT, and this was reflected in the make up of the expert panel, although some GPs who were invited were unable to attend because of work commitments.

Individuals who were invited were chosen for their clinical and/or research expertise, reputation and interest. Consumer representation covered the needs of adults, children and carers. It was decided to limit the numbers of delegates (including the project team) to approximately 30 in order to facilitate discussion and the achievement of consensus.

Relevant professional organisations that were not invited were informed about the conference, advised of those attending and invited to comment on the draft guidelines.

The expert panel was present at the conference and was consulted at each stage in the development of the guidelines.

Literature review methodology

This methodology for the literature review was explained in Chapter 4.

Conference arrangements

A 2-day consensus conference was held in January 1995 for approximately 30 delegates. Prior to the conference, delegates were sent a systematic review of the literature on incontinence, an overview of the consensus conference approach and details of the questions to be discussed during the conference. The literature review prepared for the project was available at the conference.

Delegates were divided into three predetermined syndicate groups, which ensured an adequate balance of professions and interests. Members of the Steering Group facilitated the groups, and there were note-takers present throughout the conference and in each syndicate group.

The conference consisted of an overview of research into incontinence, plus the background to the project. Small group discussions were then held in the syndicate groups around predetermined questions. The discussion groups focused on:

- the definition of incontinence;
- assessment and referral;

- the promotion of continence;
- the management of incontinence;
- enuresis in children;
- faecal incontinence;
- educational issues;
- continuous quality improvement issues.

During the discussions, reference was made to the summaries of consensus within the literature review.

During plenary sessions, feedback was given from each group. Following discussions of each group's feedback, statements were produced that reflected the views of conference. These were presented on acetates to the conference for discussion and amendment. A series of consensus statements was therefore produced by the end of the conference.

Consensus agreement with statements was demonstrated by a show of hands during the conference. Anonymous written evaluations at the end of the conference asked questions regarding agreement with the statements. The results were as follows:

- 75% of the delegates said that the consensus statements produced by the conference *always* reflected their views.
- 25% said that the statements *sometimes* reflected their views.

The guidelines

The notes taken and flip charts used were analysed after the conference to confirm or clarify statements. The statements were then refined and cross-referenced with the literature review and other policy and practice guidelines to provide evidence-based rationales. The draft guidelines were then sent to the delegates for comments.

Comments were received from two-thirds of the delegates, and these were incorporated into the guidelines, directed by the following principles:

- Comments and amendments should be incorporated if at all possible.
- The intent of the consensus statements should not alter.
- The incorporation of comments should not contradict the results of the literature review.
- The consensus view should not be altered.

- The comments of delegates who attended the conference should take precedence over those of non-attenders.

The Steering Group discussed the comments received and amendments made, and the second draft of the guidelines were then sent for consultation to relevant professional groups who had agreed to comment, and to other interested parties, for their comments.

Comments were received from three-quarters of the professional groups consulted. Further amendments were then made to the guidelines as a result of these comments, using the same guiding principles and taking account of the remaining timescale for the project.

Implementation

The guidelines initially were implemented and evaluated by the project team at Castlefields Health Centre, Runcorn, Cheshire (Button *et al.*, 1996).

Glossary of terms

(Adapted from AHCPR, 1992).

Absorbent products: Pads and garments, either disposable or reusable, worn and/or placed under the patient to absorb uncontrolled urine flow.

Alarm therapy: A conditioning therapy used for nocturnal enuresis in adults and children. An electronic alarm consists of a metal sensor that is body-worn or in a mattress pad. When the sensor is moistened by urine, an electrical circuit is completed and an effector, a bell or buzzer, sounds. The device signals urination. The person eventually comes to learn the association between sensation of bladder fullness, the sounding of the alarm and the need to awaken and inhibit urination.

Behavioural techniques: Specific interventions designed to alter the relationship between the patient's symptoms and his or her environment for the treatment of maladaptive urinary voiding patterns. This may be achieved by modification of the behaviour and/or environment of the patient (see biofeedback, bladder training, electrical stimulation, habit training, pelvic muscle exercises and prompted voiding).

Benign prostatic hyperplasia (BPH): A common disorder of men over the age of 50 characterised by enlargement of the prostate, which may press against the urethra and obstruct the flow of urine. BPH is the most common cause of such anatomical obstruction in elderly men.

Biofeedback: A behavioural technique by which information about a normally unconscious physiologic process is presented to the patient and the therapist as a visual, auditory or tactile signal. The signal is derived from a measurable physiological parameter that is subsequently used in an educational process to accomplish a specific therapeutic result. The signal is displayed in a quantitative way, and the patient is taught how to alter it and thus control the physiological process.

Bladder training: A behavioural technique that requires the patient to resist or inhibit the sensation of urgency (the strong desire to urinate), to postpone voiding and to urinate according to a timetable rather than the urge to void.

Catheterisation: Techniques for managing urinary incontinence that involve the use of a slender tube inserted through the urethra or through the anterior abdominal wall into the bladder, urinary reservoir or urinary conduit to allow urine drainage.

Clinical practice guidelines: A set of systematically developed statements or recommendations designed to assist practitioner and patient decisions about appropriate health care for specific clinical circumstances. Such guidelines are designed to assist health care practitioners in the prevention, diagnosis, treatment and management of specific clinical conditions.

Colonoscopy: Endoscopic examination of the colon, either transabdominally during laparotomy or transanally by means of a colonoscope.

Cystometry: A test used to assess the function of the bladder by measuring the pressure–volume relationship of the bladder. Cystometry is used to assess detrusor activity, sensation, capacity and compliance. There are different variations of the test depending on the problem being investigated, but, regardless of the technique, cystometry involves the insertion of a catheter into the bladder.

Detrusor: A general term for any part of the body that pushes down. In the urinary system, the detrusor muscle is the smooth muscle in the wall of the urinary bladder that contracts the bladder and expels the urine.

Detrusor instability (unstable bladder): Involuntary detrusor contraction in the absence of associated neurological disorders (see urge incontinence).

Dry-bed training: This conditioning method for children with nocturnal enuresis requires the child to rehearse before bedtime the exact performance of getting out of bed, switching off the enuretic alarm, voiding in the toilet, changing the nightclothes and bedding and resetting the alarm.

Electrical stimulation: The application of an electric current to stimulate or inhibit the pelvis viscera or their nerve supply in order to directly induce a therapeutic response.

Encopresis: Incontinence of faeces not arising from organic defect or illness.

Enuresis: The involuntary discharge of urine by day or night, or both, in a child aged 5 years or older, in the absence of congenital or acquired defects of the nervous system or urinary tract (Forsythe and Butler, 1989).

Faecal impaction: Accumulation of putty-like or hardened faeces in the rectum or sigmoid colon.

Faecal occult blood: Examination, microscopically or by a chemical test, of a specimen of faeces to determine the presence of blood not otherwise detectable.

Frequency: Urination at short intervals without an increase in daily volume of urinary output.

Frequency–volume chart: A record maintained by the patient or caregiver that is used to record the frequency, timing, amount of voiding and/or other factors associated with the patient's urinary incontinence.

Genuine stress incontinence: The condition in which involuntary loss of urine occurs when, in the absence of a detrusor contraction, the intravesical pressure exceeds the maximum urethral pressure.

Habit training: A behavioural technique in which the time between voiding is altered to suit the individual's voiding pattern, either increased or decreased.

Hyperreflexia: Any exaggeration of reflexes. In urinary incontinence, an involuntary detrusor contraction resulting from a neurological disorder.

Incidence: The number of particular *new* cases of a condition occurring in a population in a given period of time.

Incontinence: A condition in which the involuntary loss of urine or faeces is a social or hygienic problem.

Indwelling catheters: Tube devices inserted into the bladder, urinary reservoir or urinary conduit for a period of time longer than one emptying.

Intermittent catheterisation: The use of a catheter inserted through the urethra into the bladder at regular intervals for bladder drainage, being removed each time.

Involuntary detrusor contraction: A cause of urinary incontinence resulting from uncontrolled contractions of the detrusor.

Mixed urinary incontinence: The combination in a patient of urge urinary incontinence and stress urinary incontinence.

Nocturnal enuresis: The involuntary loss of urine (urinary incontinence) during sleep. Also called bedwetting. May occur in adults and children.

Overactive bladder: A condition characterised by involuntary detrusor contractions during the bladder-filling phase, which may be spontaneous or provoked and which the patient cannot suppress.

Overflow incontinence: The involuntary loss of urine associated with overdistension of the bladder. Overflow incontinence results from urinary retention that causes the capacity of the bladder to be overwhelmed. Continuous or intermittent leakage of a small amount of urine results.

Overlearning therapy: A conditioning method used with children suffering from nocturnal enuresis. It involves the child maintaining full nocturnal bladder control in the face of a large intake of fluid during the evening while an enuretic alarm is being used.

Pelvic muscle exercise: A behavioural technique that requires repetitive active exercise of the pubococcygeus muscle to improve urethral resistance and urinary control by strengthening the peri-urethral and pelvic muscles. Also called Kegel exercises in American literature.

Penile sheaths: Devices for externally draining the bladder, made from latex rubber, polyvinyl or silicone, that are secured on the shaft of the penis by some form of adhesive and are connected to urine-collecting bags by a tube.

Pessaries: Devices for women that are placed intravaginally to treat pelvic relaxation or prolapse of pelvic organs.

Post-voiding residual (PVR) volume: The amount of fluid remaining in the bladder immediately following the completion of urination. Estimation of PVR volume can be made by abdominal palpation and percussion or bimanual examination. Specific measurement of PVR volume can be accomplished by catheterisation, pelvic ultrasound, radiography or radioisotope studies.

Prevalence: The total number of cases of a specific disease or condition in existence in a given population at a certain time.

Primary health care team (PHCT): An extended team of GPs, attached and employed nurses, other health care workers and administrative staff, servicing a defined population, having easier patient access and more comprehensive medical information about each patient than other parts of the NHS.

Prompted voiding: A behavioural technique for use primarily with dependent or cognitively impaired persons. Prompted voiding attempts to teach the incontinent person awareness of his or her incontinence status and to request toileting assistance, either independently or after being prompted by a caregiver.

Provocative stress test: A test to confirm stress urinary incontinence, performed by having the patient relax and then cough vigorously while the examiner observes for urine loss from the urethra. Ideally, the patient's bladder should be full, but the test should not be performed when the patient has a precipitant urge to void. The patient can be standing or in the lithotomy position. If an instantaneous leakage occurs with cough, stress incontinence is likely; if leakage is delayed or persists after the cough, detrusor overactivity should be suspected. If the test is initially performed in the lithotomy position and no leakage is observed, the test should be repeated in the standing position.

Sensory urgency: Urgency associated with bladder hypersensitivity (see urge/urgency).

Sigmoidoscopy: Direct examination of the interior of the sigmoid colon, up to the rectum.

Stress incontinence: A symptom of urinary incontinence characterised by the involuntary loss of urine from the urethra during physical exertion, for example during coughing.

Timed voiding: A behavioural technique that involves scheduled voiding to a rigid regime, usually with a 2-hourly interval.

Transient urinary incontinence: Temporary episodes of urinary incontinence that are reversible once the cause or causes of the episode(s) have been identified and treated.

Ultrasonography: A technique that uses ultrasound to obtain visual images of the urinary tract or anal sphincter for the purpose of assessing its anatomical status.

Underactive bladder: A condition characterised by a bladder contraction of inadequate magnitude and/or duration to effect bladder emptying in a normal timespan. This condition can be caused by drugs, faecal impaction and neurological conditions such as diabetic neuropathy or low spinal cord injury, or as a result of radical pelvic surgery. It can also result from the weakening of the detrusor muscle from vitamin B12 deficiency or idiopathic causes. Bladder underactivity may cause overdistension of the bladder, resulting in overflow incontinence (see overflow incontinence).

Urge incontinence: The involuntary loss of urine associated with an abrupt and strong desire to void (urgency). Urge incontinence is often associated with the urodynamic findings of involuntary detrusor contractions or detrusor overactivity.

Urge/urgency: A strong desire to void.

Urinary tract: Passageway from the pelvis to the kidney to the urinary orifice through the ureters, bladder and urethra.

Urodynamic tests: Tests designed to determine the anatomical and functional status of the urinary bladder and urethra.

References

ACA (Association for Continence Advice) (1993) *Guidelines for Continence Care.* London: ACA.

ACA (Association for Continence Advice) (1988) *Directory of Continence and Toileting Aids.* London: Disabled Living Foundation.

Addison R, Roe B, Taylor P (1994). *The Role of the Continence Adviser. Clinical Practice–A Principal Function.* London: RCN.

AHCPR (Agency for Health Care Policy and Research) Urinary Incontinence Guideline Panel (1992) *Urinary Incontinence in Adults: Clinical Practice Guideline.* Rockville, MD: Agency for Health Care Policy and Research, Public Health Service, US Department of Health and Human Services.

Ahlstrom K, Sandahl B, Sjoberg B, Ulmsten U, Stormby N, Lindskog M (1990) Effect of combined treatment with phenylpropanolamine and estriol, compared with estriol treatment alone, in postmenopausal women with stress urinary incontinence. *Gynecologic and Obstetric Investigation 30*(1): 37–43.

Allen RE, Hosker GL, Smith AR, Warrell DW (1990) Pelvic floor damage and childbirth: a neurophysiological study. *British Journal of Obstetrics and Gynaecology 97*(9): 770–9.

Andersen JT, Abrams P, Blaivas JG, Stanton SL (1988) The standardisation of terminology of lower urinary tract function. *Scandinavian Journal of Urology and Nephrology 114 (Suppl.):* 5–19.

Andersson KE (1988). Current concepts in the treatment of disorders of micturition. *Drugs 35*: 477–94.

Ashworth PD, Hagan MT (1993) The meaning of incontinence: a qualitative study of non-geriatric urinary incontinence sufferers. *Journal of Advanced Nursing 18*(9): 1415–23.

Bakke A, Brun OH, Hoisaeter PA (1992) Clinical background of patients treated with clean intermittent catheterization in Norway. *Scandinavian Journal of Urology and Nephrology 26*(3): 211–17.

Bakke A, Irgens LM, Malt UF, Hoisaeter PA (1993) Clean intermittent catheterisation-performing abilities, aversive experiences and distress. *Paraplegia 31*: 288–97.

Barrett JA (1992) Faecal incontinence. In Roe BH (ed.) *Clinical Nursing Practice. The Promotion and Management of Continence*. London: Prentice Hall, pp 196–219.

Barrett JA (1993) *Faecal Incontinence and Related Problems in the Older Adult*. London: Edward Arnold.

Barrett JA, Brocklehurst JC, Kiff ES, Ferguson G, Faragher EB (1990) Rectal motility studies in faecally incontinent geriatric patients. *Age and Ageing 19*, 311–17.

Bartolo DCC, Kamm MA, Kuijpers H, Lubowski MD, Pembertin JH, Rothenberger MD (1994) Working Party Report: Defecation disorders. *American Journal of Gastroenterology 89*(8): S154–S159.

Bassotti G, Whitehead W (1994) Biofeedback as a treatment approach to gastrointestinal tract disorders. *American Journal of Gastroenterology 89*(2): 158–64.

Berglund A-L, Fugl-Meyer KS (1991) Sexual problems in women with urinary incontinence. *Scandinavian Journal of Caring Sciences 5*(1): 13–16.

Bergman A, Bader K (1990) Reliability of the patient's history in the diagnosis of urinary incontinence. *International Journal of Gynaecology and Obstetrics 32*(3): 255–9.

Bernard MA (1994) Urinary incontinence in elderly females. *Journal of Oklahoma State Medical Association 87*: 217–24.

Birgersson AM Bjurbrant, Hammar V, Widersfors G, Hallberg IR (1993) Elderly women's feelings about being urinary incontinent, using napkins and being helped by nurses to change napkins. *Journal of Clinical Nursing 2*: 165–71.

Blackwell C (1995) *A Guide to Enuresis*. Bristol: ERIC.

Bloom DA, Seeley WW, Ritchley ML, McGuire EJ (1993) Toilet habits and continence in children: an opportunity sampling in search of normal parameters. *Journal of Urology 149*(5): 1087–90.

Borrie MJ, Davidson HA (1992) Incontinence in institutions: costs and contributing factors. *Canadian Medical Association Journal 147*(3): 322–8.

Brading AF, Turner WH (1994) The unstable bladder: towards a common mechanism. *British Journal of Urology 73*: 3–8.

Briggs M, Williams ES (1992) Urinary incontinence. *British Medical Journal 304*: 255.

Brink CA (1990) Absorbent pads, garments, and management strategies. *Journal of the American Geriatrics Society 38*(3): 368–73.

Brocklehurst JC (1990a) Urinary incontinence in old age: helping the general practitioner to make a diagnosis. *Gerontology 36*: 3–7.

Brocklehurst JC (1990b) Professional and public education about incontinence. The British experience. *Journal of the American Geriatrics Society 38*(3): 384–6.

Brocklehurst JC (1993) Urinary incontinence in the community–analysis of a MORI poll. *British Medical Journal 306*: 832–34.

Brocklehurst N (1994) *Purchasing for Continence Promotion. Guidelines for Health Authorities and GP Fundholders on Commissioning Continence Services*. West Midlands Regional Health Authority.

Brown C (1994) Community care. *Nursing Times 90*(4): 86–9.

Brown J, White H (1991) An incontinence helpline service. *Nursing Standard 5*(38): 25–7.

Brubaker L, Kotarinos R (1993) Kegel or cut? Variations on his theme. *Journal of Reproductive Medicine 38*(9): 672–8.

Bump RC (1993) Racial comparisons and contrasts in urinary incontinence and pelvic organ prolapse. *Obstetrics and Gynaecology 81*(3): 421–5.

Bump R, McClish DK (1992) Cigarette smoking and urinary incontinence in women. *American Journal of Obstetrics and Gynecology 167*: 1213–18.

Bump R, McClish DM (1994) Cigarette smoking and pure stress incontinence of urine: a comparison of risk factors and determinants between smokers and non-smokers. *American Journal of Obstetrics and Gynecology 170*: 579–82.

Bump R, Hurt WG, Fantl A, Wyman JF (1991) Assessment of Kegel pelvic muscle exercise after brief verbal instruction. *American Journal of Obstetrics and Gynecology 165*(2): 322–9.

Bump RC, Sugarman HJ, Fantl JA, McClish DK (1992) Obesity and lower urinary tract function in women: effect of surgically induced weight loss. *American Journal of Obstetrics and Gynecology 167*(2): 392–7.

Burgio KL (1990) Behavioral training for stress and urge incontinence in the community. *Gerontology 36*: 27–34.

Burgio KL, Matthews KA, Engel BT (1991) Prevalence, incidence and correlates of urinary incontinence in healthy, middle-aged women. *Journal of Urology 146*: 1255–9.

Burgio LD, McCormick KA, Scheve AS, Engel BT, Hawkins A, Leahy E (1994) The effects of changing prompted voiding schedules in the treatment of incontinence in nursing home residents. *Journal of the American Geriatrics Society 42*(3): 315–20.

Burnet C, Carter H, Gorman D (1992) Urinary incontinence: a survey of knowledge, working practice and training needs of nursing staff in Fife. *Health Bulletin 50*(6): 448–52.

Burns PA, Pranikoff K, Nochajski TH, Hadley EC, Levy KJ, Ory MG (1993) A comparison of effectiveness of biofeedback and pelvic muscle exercise treatment of stress incontinence in older community-dwelling women. *Journal of Gerontology 48*(4): M167–M174.

Butler RJ (1991) Establishment of working definitions in nocturnal enuresis. *Archives of Disease in Childhood 66*: 267–71.

Butler RJ (1993) *Enuresis Resource Pack: Charts, Questionnaires and Information to Assist Professionals*. Bristol: ERIC.

Butler RJ (1994) *Nocturnal Enuresis: The Child's Experience*. London: Butterworth Heinemann.

Button DE, Roe B, Webb C, Frith T, Colin-Thome D, Gardner L (1996) *The Development, Implementation and Evaluation of Consensus Guidelines for the Promotion and Management of Continence by the Primary Health Care Team*. Unpublished report to the NHSE, Leeds. Runcorn: Castlefields Health Centre.

Cammu H, Debruyne R, van Nylen M, Derde MP, Amy JJ (1991) Pelvic physiotherapy in genuine stress incontinence. *Urology 38*(4): 332–7.

Caputo RM, Benson JT (1992). Idiopathic fecal incontinence. *Current Opinions in Obstetrics and Gynaecology 4*:565–70.

Caputo RM, Benson JT, McClellan E (1993) Intravaginal maximal electrical stimulation in the treatment of urinary incontinence. *Journal of Reproductive Medicine 38*(9): 667–71.

Cardozo L (1991) Urinary incontinence in women, have we anything new to offer? *British Medical Journal 303*: 1453–7.

Cardozo L, Kelleher C (1994) Sex hormones and the female lower urinary tract. *Physiotherapy 80*(3): 135–8.

Charter for Continence (1995) Charter for Continence. Developed by Continence Foundation, InContact, ACA, RCN Continence Care Forum, ERIC, Spinal Injuries Association and Multiple Sclerosis Society. Produced by educational grant from Bard Limited.

Cheater F (1991a) Attitudes towards urinary incontinence. *Nursing Standard 20*(5): 23–7.

Cheater F (1991b) Continence training programmes: need for standardisation. *Nursing Standard 6*(8): 24–7.

Cheater F (1992) The aetiology of urinary incontinence. In Roe BH (ed.) *Clinical Nursing Practice. The Promotion and Management of Continence.* London: Prentice Hall, pp 20–48.

Clark A, Romm J (1993) Effect of urinary incontinence on sexual activity in women. *Journal of Reproductive Medicine 38*(9): 679–83.

Clark G, Fleming C, Habel A, Hindmarsh J, Hunt S, Polnay L, Thakaran M (1994) Nocturnal enuresis: a strategy for management. *Hospital Update (Suppl.)* Sep: 1–11.

Colling J, Ouslander J, Hadley BJ, Eisch J, Campbell E (1992) The effects of patterned urge response toileting (PURT) on urinary incontinence among nursing home residents. *Journal of the American Geriatrics Society 40*(2): 135–41.

Continence Foundation (1992) *Continence in Primary Care–A Resource Pack.* London: Continence Foundation.

Continence Foundation (1994) *The Continence Guide '94.* London: Continence Foundation.

Continence Foundation (1995a) *Commissioning Comprehensive Continence Services: Guidance for Purchasers.* London: Continence Foundation.

Continence Foundation (1995b) *Guidelines on Working with Ethnic Minority Communities.* London: Continence Foundation.

Corbett-Nolan A (1994) Setting standards. *Nursing Times 90*(43): 64–5.

Cottenden A (1992) Aids and appliances for incontinence. In Roe BH (ed.) *Clinical Nursing Practice. The Promotion and Management of Continence.* London: Prentice Hall, pp 127–56.

Cottenden A, Ledger D (1993) Incontinence pads: predicting their leakage performance using laboratory tests. *Neurourology and Urodynamics 12*: 289–91.

Creighton SM, Stanton SL (1990) Caffeine; does it affect your bladder? *British Journal of Urology 66*: 613–14.

Cullum N (1994) *The Nursing Management of Leg Ulcers in the Community: A Critical Review of Research.* University of Liverpool: Department of Nursing.

Cutler WB, Friedmann E, Felmet K, Genovese-Stone E (1992) Stress urinary incontinence: a pervasive problem among healthy women. *Journal of Women's Health 1*(4): 259–66.

Davila GW, Ostermann KV (1994) The bladder neck support prosthesis: a nonsurgical approach to stress incontinence in adult women. *American Journal of Obstetrics and Gynecology 171*(1): 206–10.

Dawes H (1994) Campaigning for continence care. *Nursing Standard 9*(8): 23–5.

Devlin JB (1991) Prevalence and risk factors for childhood enuresis. *Irish Medical Journal 84*: 118–20.

DH (Department of Health) (1991) *Agenda for Action on Incontinence.* London: DH.

DH (Department of Health) (1993) *A Vision for the Future.* London: DH/NHSME.

DH (Department of Health) (1995) *The Patient's Charter and You.* London: DH.

Diokno AC, Brock BM, Herzog AR, Bromberg J (1990) Medical correlates of urinary incontinence in the elderly. *Urology 36*(2): 129–38.

Diokno AC, Brown MB, Herzog AR (1991) Relationship between use of diuretics and continence status in the elderly. *Urology 38*(1): 39–42.

Dorsey JH, Cundiff G (1994) Laparoscopic procedures for incontinence and prolapse. *Current Opinion in Obstetrics and Gynecology 6*: 223–30.

Dougherty M, Bishop K, Mooney R, Gimotty P, Williams B (1993) Graded pelvic muscle exercise–effect on stress urinary incontinence. *Journal of Reproductive Medicine 38*(9): 684–91.

Dowd TT (1991) Discovering older women's experience of urinary incontinence. *Research in Nursing and Health 14*: 179–86.

Duffin H (1992) Assessment of urinary incontinence. In Roe BH (ed.) *Clinical Nursing Practice. The Promotion and Management of Continence*. London: Prentice Hall, pp 1–16.

Dwyer PL, Teele JS (1992) Prazosin: a neglected cause of genuine stress incontinence. *Obstetrics and Gynaecology 79*(1): 117–21.

Elia G, Bergman A (1993) Pelvic muscle exercises: when do they work? *Obstetrics and Gynecology 81*(2): 283–6.

Enck P (1993) Biofeedback training in disordered defecation. A critical review. *Digestive Diseases and Sciences 38*(11): 1953–60.

Engel BT, Burgio LD, McCormick K, Hawkins AM, Scheve ASS, Leahy E (1990) Behavioral treatment of incontinence in the long-term care setting. *Journal of the American Geriatrics Society 38*(3): 361–3.

ERIC (1995) *Charter for Children with Bedwetting and Daytime Wetting and Their Families*. Bristol: ERIC.

Esa A, Kiwamoto H, Sugiyama T, Park YC, Kaneko S, Kurita T (1991) Functional electrical stimulation in the management of incontinence: studies of urodynamics. *International Urology and Nephrology 23*(2): 135–41.

Fantl JA, Wyman JF, McClish DK, Karkins SW, Elswick RK, Taylor JR, Hadley EC (1991) Efficacy of bladder training in older women with urinary incontinence. *Journal of the American Medical Association 265*(5): 609–13.

Fantl JA, Cardozo L, McClish DK (1994) Estrogen therapy in the management of urinary incontinence in postmenopausal women: a meta-analysis. First report of the Hormones and Urogenital Therapy Committee. *Obstetrics and Gynecology 83*(1): 12–18.

Felt-Bersma RJF, Cuesta MA (1994) Faecal incontinence 1994: which test and which treatment? *Netherlands Journal of Medicine 44*(5): 182–8.

Flaherty JH, Miller DK, Coe RM (1992) Impact on caregivers of supporting urinary function in noninstitutionalized, chronically ill seniors. *Gerontologist 32*(4): 541–5.

Flynn L, Cell P, Luisi E (1994) Effectiveness of pelvic muscle exercises in reducing urge incontinence among community residing elders. *Journal of Gerontological Nursing 20*(5): 23–7.

Foldspang A, Mommsen S, Lam GW, Elving L (1992) Parity as a correlate of adult female urinary incontinence prevalence. *Journal of Epidemiology and Community Health 46*: 595–600.

Foldspang A, Mommsen S (1994) Adult female urinary incontinence and childhood bedwetting. *Journal of Urology 152*(1): 85–8.

Fonda D (1990) Improving management of urinary incontinence in geriatric centres and nursing homes. Victorian Geriatricians Peer Review Group. *Australian Clinical Review 10*(2): 66–71.

Forsythe WI, Butler RJ (1989) Fifty years of enuretic alarms. *Archives of Disease in Childhood 64*: 879–85.

Fossberg E, Sorensen S, Ruutu M, Bakka A, Stien R, Henriksson L, Kinn AC (1990) Maximal electrical stimulation in the treatment of unstable detrusor and urge incontinence. *European Urology 18*: 120–3.

Fultz NH, Herzog AR (1993) Measuring urinary incontinence in surveys. *Gerontologist 33*(6): 708–13.

Gelber DA, Good DC, Laven LJ, Verhulst SJ (1993) Causes of urinary incontinence after acute hemispheric stroke. *Stroke 24*(3): 378–82.

Getliffe KA (1994) The use of bladder wash-outs to reduce urinary catheter encrustation. *British Journal of Urology 73*: 696–700.

Gibb H, Wong G (1994) How to choose: nurses' judgements of the effectiveness of a range of currently marketed continence aids. *Journal of Clinical Nursing 3*: 77–86.

Goldstein M, Hawthorne ME, Engberg S, McDowell BJ, Burgio KL (1992) Urinary incontinence: why people do not seek help. *Journal of Gerontological Nursing 18*(4): 15–20.

Gould D (1994) Keeping on tract. *Nursing Times 90*(40): 58–64.

Greenfield SP, Fera M (1991) The use of intravesical oxybutynin chloride in children with neurogenic bladder. *Journal of Urology 146*(2): 532–4.

Griffiths DJ, McCracken PN, Harrison GM, Gormley EA, Moore K, Hooper R, McEwan ABJ, Triscott J (1994) Cerebral aetiology of urinary urge incontinence in elderly people. *Age and Ageing 23*: 246–50.

Grimby A, Milsom I, Molander U, Wiklund I, Ekelund P (1993) The influence of urinary incontinence on the quality of life of elderly women. *Age and Ageing 22*: 82–9.

Gustafson R (1993) Conditioning treatment of children's bedwetting: a follow-up and predictive study. *Psychological Reports 72*(3, part 1): 923–30.

Hadley EC (1986) Bladder training and related therapies for urinary incontinence in older people. *Journal of the American Medical Association 256*(3): 372–9.

Hahn I, Sommar S, Fall M (1991) A comparative study of pelvic floor training and electrical stimulation for the treatment of genuine female stress urinary incontinence. *Neurourology and Urodynamics 10*: 545–54.

Hahn I, Milsom I, Fall M, Ekelund P (1993) Long term results of pelvic floor training in female stress urinary incontinence. *British Journal of Urology 72*: 421–7.

Hallan RI, George B, Williams NS (1993) Anal sphincter function: fecal incontinence and its treatment. *Annals of the Royal College of Surgeons 25*(2): 85–115.

Hanley J (1992) Choosing garments to aid incontinence. *Nursing Times 88* (27): 50–1.

Hansson S (1992) Urinary incontinence in children and associated problems. *Scandinavian Journal of Urology and Nephrology 141 (Suppl.)*: 47–55.

Harrison GL, Memel DS (1994) Urinary incontinence in women: its prevalence and its management in a health promotion clinic. *British Journal of General Practice 44*(381): 149–52.

Hellstrom E, Ekelund P, Milsom I, Mellstrom D (1990a) The prevalence of urinary incontinence and use of incontinence aids in 85-year-old men and women. *Age and Ageing 19*(6): 383–9.

Hellstrom AL, Hanson E, Hansson S, Hjalmas K, Jodal U (1990b) Micturition habits and incontinence in 7-year-old Swedish school entrants. *European Journal of Pediatrics 149*(6): 434–7.

Hellstrom L, Ekelund P, Larsson M, Milsom I (1993) Adapting incontinent patients' incontinence aids to their leakage volumes. *Scandinavian Journal of Caring Sciences 7*: 67–71.

Herzog AR, Fultz NH (1990) Prevalence and incidence of urinary incontinence in community-dwelling populations. *Journal of the American Geriatrics Society 38*: 273–81.

Herzog AR, Diokno AC, Brown MB, Normolle DP, Brock BM (1990) Two-year incidence, remission, and change patterns of urinary incontinence in noninstitutionalised older adults. *Journal of Gerontology 45*(2): 67–74.

Herzog AR, Diokno AC, Brown MB, Fultz NH, Goldstein NE (1994) Urinary incontinence as a risk factor for mortality. *Journal of the American Geriatrics Society 42*(3): 264–8.

Horgan AF, Prasad B, Waldron DJ, O'Sullivan DC (1992) Acute urinary retention. Comparison of suprapubic and urethral catheterisation. *British Journal of Urology* 70: 149–51.

Houston KA (1993) Incontinence and the older woman. *Clinics in Geriatric Medicine 9*: 157–71.

Hu T (1990) Impact of urinary incontinence on health-care costs. *Journal of the American Geriatrics Society 38*(3): 292–5.

Humphris D (1994) Clinical guidelines: an industry for growth. *Nursing Times 90*(40): 46–7.

Hunskaar S (1992) One hundred and fifty men with urinary incontinence. *Scandinavian Journal of Primary Health Care 10*: 26–9.

Hunskaar S, Sandvik H (1993) One hundred and fifty men with urinary incontinence. *Scandinavian Journal of Primary Health Care 11*: 193–6.

Hunskaar S, Vinsnes A (1991) The quality of life in women with urinary incontinence as measured by the sickness impact profile. *Journal of the American Geriatrics Society 39*(4): 378–92.

Hyland N (1991) Training for success. *Nursing Times 87*(32): 61–2.

Jarvis GJ (1994) Surgery for genuine stress incontinence. *British Journal of Obstetrics and Gynaecology 10*: 371–4.

Jensen JK, Nielsen FR, Ostergard DR (1994) The role of patient history in the diagnosis of urinary incontinence. *Obstetrics and Gynecology 83*(5): 904–10.

Jeter KF, Wagner DB (1990) Incontinence in the American home: a survey of 36,500 people. *Journal of the American Geriatrics Society 38*(3): 379–83.

Jolleys JV (1988) Reported prevalence of urinary incontinence in women in a general practice. *British Medical Journal 296*: 1300–2.

Jolleys J, Wilson J (1993) GPs lack confidence. *British Medical Journal 306*: 1344.

Jorge JMN, Wexner SD (1993) Etiology and management of fecal incontinence. *Diseases of the Colon and Rectum 36*(1): 77–97.

Ju CC, Swan LK, Merriman A, Choon TE, Viegas O (1991) Urinary incontinence among the elderly people of Singapore. *Age and Ageing 20*(4): 262–6.

Kennedy A (1992) Bladder re-education for the promotion of continence. In Roe BH (ed.) *Clinical Nursing Practice. The Promotion and Management of Continence.* London: Prentice Hall, pp 75–94.

Kinn AC, Larsson PO (1990) Desmopressin: a new principle for symptomatic treatment of urgency incontinence in patients with multiple sclerosis. *Scandinavian Journal of Urology and Nephrology 24*(2): 109–12.

Klemm LW, Creason NS (1991) Self-care practices of women with urinary incontinence–a preliminary study. *Health Care for Women International 12*: 199–209.

Knight SJ, Laycock J (1994) The role of biofeedback in pelvic floor re-education. *Physiotherapy 80*(3): 145–8.

Kok AL, Voorhorst FJ, Burger CW, van-Houten P, Kenemans P (1992) Urinary and faecal incontinence in community-residing elderly women. *Age and Ageing 21*(3): 211–15.

Lagace EA, Hansen W, Hickner JM (1993) Prevalence and severity of urinary incontinence in ambulatory adults: a UPRNet study. *Journal of Family Practice 36*(6): 610–14.

Lagro-Janssen TLM, Smits AJA, van Weel C (1990) Women with urinary incontinence: self-perceived worries and general practitioner's knowledge of problem. *British Journal of General Practice 40*: 331–4.

Lagro-Janssen TLM, Debruyne FMJ, Smits AJA, van Weel C (1991) Controlled trial of pelvic floor exercises in the treatment of urinary stress incontinence in general practice. *British Journal of General Practice 41*: 445–9.

Lagro-Janssen ALM, Debruyne FMJ, van Weel C (1991) Value of the patient's case history in diagnosing urinary incontinence in general practice. *British Journal of Urology 67*: 569–72.

Lagro-Janssen ALM, Debruyne FMJ, van Weel C (1992) Psychological aspects of female urinary incontinence in general practice. *British Journal of Urology 70*: 499–502.

Lagro-Janssen T, Smits A, van Weel C (1992) Urinary incontinence in women and the effects on their lives. *Scandinavian Journal of Primary Health Care 10*: 211–16.

Lagro-Janssen ALM, Debruyne FMJ, Smits AJA, van Weel C (1992) The effects of treatment of urinary incontinence in general practice. *Family Practice 9*(3): 284–9.

Lam GW, Foldspang A, Elving LB, Mommsen S (1992) Social context, social abstention, and problem recognition correlated with adult female urinary incontinence. *Danish Medical Bulletin 39*(6): 565–70.

Laycock J (1992) Pelvic floor re-education for the promotion of continence. In Roe BH (ed.) *Clinical Nursing Practice. The Promotion and Management of Continence.* London: Prentice Hall, pp 95–126.

Laycock J (1995) Must do better. *Nursing Times 91*(7): 64.

Laycock J, Jerwood D (1994) Development of the Bradford perineometer. *Physiotherapy 80*(3): 139–42.

LeCoutour X, Jung-Faerber S, Klein P, Renaud R (1990) Female urinary incontinence: comparative value of history and urodynamic investigations. *European Journal of Obstetrics and Gynecology and Reproductive Biology 37*: 279–86.

Lindehall B, Moller A, Hjalmas K, Jodal U (1994) Long-term intermittent catheterization: the experience of teenagers and young adults with myelomeningocele. *Journal of Urology 152*(1): 187–9.

Lin-Dyken DC, Wolraich ML, Hawtrey CE, Doja MS (1992) Follow-up of clean intermittent catheterization for children with neurogenic bladders. *Urology 40*(6): 525–9.

Macaulay AJ, Stern RS, Stanton SL (1991) Psychological aspects of 211 female patients attending a urodynamic unit. *Journal of Psychosomatic Research 35*(1): 1–10.

McClish DK, Fantl JA, Wyman JF, Pisani G, Bump RC (1991) Bladder training in older women with urinary incontinence: relationship between outcome and changes in urodynamic observations. *Obstetrics and Gynecology 77*(2): 281–6.

McCormick KA, Burgio LD, Engel BT, Scheve A, Leahy E (1992) Urinary incontinence: an augmented prompted void approach. *Journal of Gerontological Nursing 18*(3): 3–10.

McDowell BJ, Burgio KL, Dombrowski M, Locher JL, Rodriguez E (1992) An interdisciplinary approach to the assessment and behavioral treatment of urinary incontinence in geriatric outpatients. *Journal of the American Geriatrics Society 40*(4): 370–4.

McGrother CW, Jagger C, Clarke M, Castleden CM (1990) Handicaps associated with incontinence: implications for management. *Journal of Epidemiology and Community Health 44*: 246–8.

McKeever MP (1990) An investigation of recognized incontinence within a health authority. *Journal of Advanced Nursing 15*: 1197–1207.

Maizels M, Gandhi K, Keating B, Rosenbaum D (1993) Diagnosis and treatment for children who cannot control urination. *Current Problems in Pediatrics* Nov/Dec: 402–51.

Malone-Lee J (1994) Recent developments in urinary incontinence in late life. *Physiotherapy 80*(3): 133–4.

Mantle J, Versi E (1991) Physiotherapy for stress urinary incontinence: a national survey. *British Medical Journal 302*: 753–5.

Meadows SR (1990) Day wetting. *Paediatric Nephrology 4*: 178–84.

Menon EB, Tan ES (1992) Bladder training in patients with spinal cord injury. *Urology 40*(5):425–9.

Meyer S, Dhenin T, Schmidt N, De Grandi P (1992) Subjective and objective effects of intravaginal electrical myostimulation and biofeedback in patients with genuine stress urinary incontinence. *British Journal of Urology 69*: 584–8.

Mizunaga M, Miyata M, Kaneko S, Yachiku S, Chiba K (1994) Intravesical instillation of oxybutinin hydrochloride therapy for patients with a neuropathic bladder. *Paraplegia 32*(1): 25–9.

Moffat MEK, Harlos S, Kirshen AJ, Burd L (1993) Desmopressin acetate and nocturnal enuresis: how much do we know? *Pediatrics 92*(3): 420–5.

Mohide EA (1992) The prevalence of urinary incontinence. In Roe BH (ed.) *Clinical Nursing Practice: The Promotion and Management of Continence*. London: Prentice Hall, pp 1–19.

Molander U (1993) Urinary incontinence and related urogenital symptoms in elderly women. *Acta Obstetricia et Gynecologica Scandinavica 72*: 5–22.

Mommsen S, Foldspang A, Elving L, Lam GW (1993) Association between urinary incontinence in women and a previous history of surgery. *British Journal of Urology 72*: 30–7.

Moore K, Richmond DH, Parys BT (1991) Sex distribution of adult idiopathic detrusor instability in relation to childhood bedwetting. *British Journal of Urology 68*: 479–82.

Moore KH, Sutherst JR (1990) Response to treatment of detrusor instability in relation to psychoneurotic status. *British Journal of Urology 66*: 486–90.

Moore KN (1994) Electrical stimulation for the treatment of urinary incontinence: do we know enough to accept it as part of our practice? *Journal of Advanced Nursing 20*: 1018–22.

Morgan R (1993) *Guidelines on Minimum Standards of Practice in the Treatment of Enuresis*. Bristol: ERIC.

Morrison LM, Glen ES, Cherry LC, Dawes H (1992) The Open Access Continence Resource Centre for Greater Glasgow Health Board. *British Journal of Urology 70*: 395–8.

Mouritsen L, Frimodt-Moller C, Moller M (1991) Long-term effect of pelvic floor exercises on female urinary incontinence. *British Journal of Urology 68*: 32–7.

Mulrow CD (1987) The medical review article: state of the science. *Annals of Internal Medicine 106*: 485–8.

NHS Executive (1995) *Incontinence–Patients' Perceptions of Services*. Leeds: NHS Executive.

NHS Management Executive (1993) Priorities and Planning Guidance 1994–5. EL (93) 54. Leeds: Department of Health.

Norgaard JP, Djurhuus JC (1993) The pathophysiology of enuresis in children and young adults. *Clinical Pediatrics (Philadelphia) Special Number*. 5–9.

Norris C, Cottenden A, Ledger D (1993) Underpad overview. *Nursing Times 89*(21): 68–74.

North A (1994) The client's view. *Nursing Times 90*(4): 80–2.

Norton C (1986) *Nursing for Continence*. Beaconsfield: Beaconsfield Publishers.

Norton KRW, Bhat AV, Stanton SL (1990) Psychiatric aspects of urinary incontinence in women attending at outpatient urodynamic clinic. *British Medical
Journal 301*: 271–2.

Nygaard I, DeLancey JO, Arnsdorf L (1990) Exercise and incontinence. *Obstetrics
and Gynecology 75*(5): 848–51.

Nygaard IE, Thompson FL, Svengalis SL, Albright JP (1994) Urinary incontinence
in elite nulliparous women. *Obstetrics and Gynecology 84*(2): 183–7.

Oakeshott P, Hunt GM (1992) Intermittent self catheterization for patients with
urinary incontinence or difficulty emptying the bladder. *British Journal of General
Practice 42*: 253–5.

O'Brien J, Austin M, Sethi P, O'Boyle P (1991) Urinary incontinence: prevalence,
need for treatment, and effectiveness of intervention by nurse. *British Medical
Journal 303*: 1308–12.

O'Donnell PD, Doyle R (1991) Biofeedback therapy technique for treatment of urinary incontinence. *Urology 37*(5): 432–6.

O'Donnell BF, Drachman DA, Barnes HJ, Peterson KE, Swearer JM, Lew RA
(1992) Incontinence and troublesome behaviors predict institutionalization in
dementia. *Journal of Geriatric Psychiatry and Neurology 5*: 45–52.

Ouslander JG, Abelson S (1990) Perceptions of urinary incontinence among elderly
outpatients. *Gerontologist 30*(3): 369–72.

Ouslander JG, Zarit SH, Orr NK, Muira SA (1990) Incontinence among elderly
community-dwelling dementia patients. *Journal of the American Geriatrics Society
38*(4): 440–5.

Ouslander JG, Palmer MH, Rovner BW, German PS (1993) Urinary incontinence
in nursing homes: incidence remission and associated factors. *Journal of the
American Geriatrics Society 41*(10): 1083–9.

Palmer MH, German PS, Ouslander JG (1991) Risk factors for urinary incontinence one year after nursing home admission. *Research in Nursing and Health 14*:
405–12.

Peattie AB, Plevnik S, Stanton SL (1988) Vaginal cones: a conservative method of
treating genuine stress incontinence. *British Journal of Obstetrics and Gynaecology 95*:
1049–53.

Philp J, Cottenden A, Ledger D (1992) The reuser's guide. *Nursing Times 88*(44):
66–72.

Philp J, Cottenden A, Ledger D (1993) Mix and match. *Nursing Times 89*(16): 70–4.

Pieper B, Cleland V (1993) An external urine-collecting device for women: a clinical trial. *Journal of ET Nursing 20*(2): 51–5.

Prasad KV, Vaidyanathan S (1993) Intravesical oxybutynin chloride and clean
intermittent catheterisation in patients with neurogenic vesical dysfunction and
decreased bladder capacity. *British Journal of Urology 72*: 719–22.

Rappaport L (1993) The treatment of nocturnal enuresis–where are we now?
Pediatrics 92(3): 465–6.

RCP (Royal College of Physicians) (1995) *Incontinence: Causes, Management and
Provision of Services. Report of the Royal College of Physicians*. London: RCP.

RCP Research Unit (1992) *The CARE Scheme: Clinical Audit of Long Term Care of Elderly
People*. London: RCP.

Rekers H, Drogendijk AC, Valkenburg H, Riphagen F (1992) Urinary incontinence in women from 35 to 79 years of age: prevalence and consequences.
European Journal of Obstetrics, Gynecology and Reproductive Biology 43: 229–34.

Resnick NM (1990a) Initial evaluation of the incontinent patient. *Journal of the
American Geriatrics Society 38*(3): 311–16.

Resnick NM (1990b) Noninvasive diagnosis of the patient with complex incontinence. *Gerontology 36*: 8–18.

Revord JP, Opitz JL, Murtaugh P, Harrison J (1993) Determining residual urine volumes using a portable ultrasonographic device. *Archives of Physical Medicine and Rehabilitation 74*: 457–62.

Reymert J, Hunskaar S (1994) Why do only a minority of perimenopausal women with urinary incontinence consult a doctor? *Scandinavian Journal of Primary Health Care 12*: 180–3.

Rhodes P (1994) Continence advisers' role in education. *Nursing Standard 8*(30): 47–53.

Rhodes P, Parker G (1993) *The Role of Continence Advisers in England and Wales*. University of York: Social Policy Research Unit.

Roe B (ed.) (1992a) *Clinical Nursing Practice: The Promotion and Management of Continence*. London: Prentice Hall.

Roe BH (1992b) Teaching patients and carers about continence. In Roe BH (ed.) *Clinical Nursing Practice: The Promotion and Management of Continence*. London: Prentice Hall, pp 231–47.

Roe BH (1992c) Use of indwelling catheters. In Roe BH (ed.) *Clinical Nursing Practice. The Promotion and Management of Continence*. London: Prentice Hall, pp 177–95.

Roe B (1993) Catheter-associated urinary tract infection: a review. *Journal of Clinical Nursing 2*: 197–203.

Roe B, Williams K (1994) *Clinical Handbook for Continence Care*. London: Scutari Press.

Roe B, Addison R, Clayton J (1992) *The Role of the Continence Adviser* London: RCN.

Rooney M (1994) Impacting health care: study of a reusable urinary drainage system. *SCI-Nursing 11*(1): 16–18.

Rushton HG (1993) Evaluation of the enuretic child. *Clinical Pediatrics (Philadelphia) Special Number.* 14–18.

Ryan-Woolley B (1987) *Aids for the Management of Incontinence*. London: King's Fund.

Sandvik H, Hunskaar S, Eriksen BJ (1990) Management of urinary incontinence in women in general practice: Actions taken at the first consultation. *Scandinavian Journal of Primary Health Care 8*: 3–8.

Sandvik H, Kveine E, Hunskaar S (1993a) Female urinary incontinence psychosocial impact, self-care, and consultations. *Scandinavian Journal of Caring Sciences 7*: 53–6.

Sandvik H, Hunskaar S, Seim A, Hermstad R, Vanvi KA, Bratt H (1993b) Validation of a severity index in female urinary incontinence and its implementation in an epidemiological survey. *Journal of Epidemiology and Community Health 47*: 497–9.

Scheuer M, Kuijpers HC, Bleijenberg G (1994) Effect of electrostimulation on sphincter function in neurogenic fecal continence. *Diseases of the Colon and Rectum 37*(6): 590–2.

Schiotz HA (1994) One month maximal electrostimulation for genuine stress incontinence in women. *Neurourology and Urodynamics 13*: 43–50.

Schneider MS, King LR, Surwit RS (1994) Kegel exercises and childhood incontinence: a new role for an old treatment. *Journal of Pediatrics 124*: 91–2.

Schnelle JF (1990) Treatment of urinary incontinence in nursing home patients by prompted voiding. *Journal of the American Geriatrics Society 38*(3): 356–60.

SE Thames RHA (1994) *Standards for Continence Advisory Services. Report from a Working Party of the SE Thames Continence Advisers Group*. Bexhill on Sea: SE Thames Regional Health Authority.

Simeonova Z, Bengtsson C (1990) Prevalence of urinary incontinence among women at a Swedish primary health care centre. *Scandinavian Journal of Primary Health Care 8*(4): 203–6.

Skoner MM, Haylor MJ (1993) Managing incontinence: women's normalizing strategies. *Health Care for Women International 14*: 549–60.

Sleep J, Grant A (1987) Pelvic floor exercises in post natal care. *Midwifery 3*: 158–64.

Smith JP (1982) *The Problems of Promoting Continence.* London: RCN and Squibb Surgicare.

Smith PS, Smith LJ (1987) *Continence and Incontinence: Psychological Approaches to Development and Treatment.* London: Croom Helm.

Smith LJ, Smith PS (1993) Psychological aspects of faecal incontinence in the elderly. In Barrett JA (ed.) *Faecal Incontinence and Related Problems in the Older Adult.* London: Edward Arnold, pp 173–206.

Smith N, Clamp M (1991) *Continence Promotion in General Practice.* Oxford: Oxford University Press.

Summitt R, Stovall TG, Bent AE, Ostergard DR (1992) Urinary incontinence: correlation of history and brief office evaluation with multichannel urodynamic testing. *American Journal of Obstetrics and Gynecology 166*(6): 1835–44.

Swaffield J (1994) The management and development of continence services within the framework of the NHS and Community Care Act (1990). *Journal of Clinical Nursing 3*: 119–24.

Swash M (1993) Faecal incontinence. *British Medical Journal 307*: 636–7.

Swithinbank LV, Carr JC, Abrams PH (1994) Longitudinal study of urinary symptoms in children. *Scandinavian Journal of Urology and Nephrology 163 (Suppl.)*: 67–73.

Szonyi G, Millard RJ (1994) Controlled trial evaluation of a general practitioner education package on incontinence: use of a mailed questionnaire. *British Journal of Urology 73*: 615–20.

Thomas AM, Morse JM (1991) Managing urinary incontinence with self-care practices. *Journal of Gerontological Nursing 17*(6): 9–14.

Thomas TM, Plymat KR, Blannin J, Meade TW (1980) Prevalence of urinary incontinence. *British Medical Journal 281*: 1243–5.

Thomas TM, Egan M, Walgrove A, Meade TW (1984) The prevalence of faecal and double incontinence. *Community Medicine 6*(3): 216–20.

Thornburn P, Cottenden A, Ledger D (1992) Undercover trials. *Nursing Times 88*(13): 72–5.

Turner-Stokes L, Frank AO (1992) Urinary incontinence among patients with arthritis–a neglected disability. *Journal of Rehabilitation and Social Medicine 85*(7): 389–93.

Vandoni RE, Lironi A, Tscantz P (1994) Bacteriuria during urinary tract catheterisation: suprapubic versus urethral route: a prospective randomized trial. *Acta Chirgica Belgique 94*(1): 12–16.

van Londen A, van Londen-Barentsen MW, van Son MJ, Mulder GA (1993) Arousal training for children suffering from nocturnal enuresis: a 2½ year follow-up. *Behavioural Research and Therapy 31*: 613–15.

Versi E, Cardozo L, Anand D, Cooper D (1991) Symptoms analysis for the diagnosis of genuine stress incontinence. *British Journal of Obstetrics and Gynaecology 98*: 815–19.

Vierhout ME, Gianotten WL (1993) Mechanisms of urine loss during sexual activity. *European Journal of Obstetrics, Gynecology and Reproductive Biology 52*(1): 45–7.

Viktrup L, Lose G, Rolff M, Barfoed K (1992) The symptom of stress incontinence caused by pregnancy or delivery in primiparas. *Obstetrics and Gynecology 79*(6): 945–9.

Vinsnes AG, Hunskaar S (1991) Distress associated with urinary incontinence, as measured by a visual analogue scale. *Scandinavian Journal of Caring Sciences* 5(1): 57–61.

Wall LL (1990) Diagnosis and management of urinary incontinence due to detrusor instability. *Obstetrical and Gynecological Survey* 45(11): 1S–47S.

Walters MD, Realini JP (1992) The evaluation and treatment of urinary incontinence in women: a primary care approach. *Journal of the American Board of Family Practitioners* 5(3): 289–301.

Walters MD, Taylor S, Schoenfeld LS (1990) Psychosexual study of women with detrusor instability. *Obstetrics and Gynecology* 75(1): 22–6.

Weese DL, Roskamp DA, Leach GE, Zimmern PE (1993) Intravesical oxybutinin chloride: experience with 42 patients. *Urology* 41(6): 527–30.

Weider DJ, Sateia MJ, West RP (1991) Nocturnal enuresis in children with upper airway obstruction. *Otolaryngology and Head and Neck Surgery* 105(3): 427–32.

Wein AJ (1990) Pharmacologic treatment of incontinence. *Journal of the American Geriatrics Society* 38(3): 317–25.

Wells T, Brink CA, Diokno AC, Wolfe R, Gillis GL (1991) Pelvic muscle exercise for stress urinary incontinence in elderly women. *Journal of the American Geriatric Society* 39: 785–791.

Williams K, Roe B (1994) *Incontinence: A Systematic Review of the Literature*. Unpublished document. Oxford: National Institute for Nursing.

Williams K, Roe B, Sindhu F (1995) *An Evaluation of Nursing Developments in Continence Care*. Oxford: National Institute for Nursing.

Winder A (1992) Intermittent self catheterisation. In Roe BH (ed.) *Clinical Nursing Practice. The Promotion and Management of Continence* (1st edn). London: Prentice Hall, pp 157–176.

Wolfs GG MC, Knottnerus JA, Janknegt RA (1994) Prevalence and detection of micturition problems among 2734 elderly men. *Journal of Urology* 152: 1467–70.

Wyman JF, Harkins SW, Fantl JA (1990) Psychosocial impact of urinary incontinence in the community-dwelling population. *Journal of the American Geriatrics Society* 38(3): 282–8.

Wyman JF, Elswick JR, Ory MG, Wilson MS, Fantl A (1993) Influence of functional, urological, and environmental characteristics on urinary incontinence in community dwelling older women. *Nursing Research* 42(5): 270–5.

Zöllner-Nielsen M, Samuelsson SM (1992) Maximal electrical stimulation of patients with frequency, urgency and urge incontinence. *Acta Obstetricia et Gynecologica Scandinavica* 71: 629–31.

Index

139